REVEALING PSYCHIATRY... FROM AN INSIDER

Revealing Psychiatry... From an Insider

Psychiatric stories for open minds and to open minds

PAVLOS SAKKAS, M.D.

Second Edition
Copyright © 2015-2023 Pavlos Sakkas
All rights reserved.

REVEALING PSYCHIATRY... FROM AN INSIDER
Psychiatric stories for open minds and to open minds
Copyright © 2015-2023 Pavlos Sakkas

Covered by Constantine Leftheriotis
Translation by Doolie Sloman
Editing by Kayleigh Hames
Photography by Efstratios Chavalezis
Illustrations (interior) by Dreamstime.com and freeicons.io
ISBN-13: 978-1-910370-73-5 (assigned to Stergiou Limited)
ePub ISBN-13: 978-1-910370-74-2 (assigned to Stergiou Limited)

First edition, 2015
Stergiou Limited, UK

Second edition (Enchanced), 2023
Stergiou Books Limited
71 Baggot Street Lower, Dublin 2, D02 P593, Ireland
Web: stergioubooks.com

Stergiou Limited is an imprint of Stergiou Books Limited
All rights reserved.

No part of this book may be reproduced in any form by any electronic or mechanical means including photocopying, recording, or information storage and retrieval without permission in writing from the author or the publisher.

DEDICATION

To my patients
and to my teachers…
Conspicuous and inconspicuous.

CONTENTS

DEDICATION	5
AUTHOR'S BIOGRAPHY	11
A FEW WORDS ABOUT THE BOOK	13
INTRODUCTION	15
THE HUMAN BRAIN: AN ADMIRABLE COMPUTER	19
Memory	19
Search engine	21
Plasticity: a gift as well as a jail	22
Habit: a gift to burn your fingers	24
The Hardware and Software in Our Brains	25
SCHIZOPHRENIA: A TINY SHORT-CIRCUIT	28
Schizophrenia: a biological illness	42
An interesting model	44
THE PATIENT'S COMPLIANCE AND HIS/HER PERSONAL RESPONSIBILITY	46
DEPRESSION: THE BATTERY NEEDS RECHARGING	48
Depression: a gift from modern life	52
RECESSION AND DEPRESSION	54
MANIA: A DATA STORM	64
Hypomania	72
ANXIETY AND PANIC ATTACKS: A USELESS ALARM SYSTEM	75
Anxiety's prehistory	75
Modern anxiety	80

The mechanism of anxiety	82
Control of the Anxiety	83
The usefulness of anxiety	84
The impact of anxiety	85
A piece of advice	86
The relation between anxiety and depression	87
The treatment for anxiety in five steps	90
OBSESSIONS AND COMPULSIONS: DEFICIENCY OF PROGRAMME LOADING	**96**
The treatment	102
DEMENTIA: AN UNAVOIDABLE DETERIORATION?	**106**
The symptoms	109
The treatment	112
SLEEP: AN OBLIGATORY 'RESTART'	**117**
The architecture of sleep	119
Dreams	119
Insomnia	121
10 recommendations for those who suffer from insomnia	124
The environment of sleep	125
ANOREXIA NERVOSA	**126**
Extreme anorexia: a programme for extreme situations	130
RESTRAINT	**134**
Addictions: stuck in a useless programme	138
An innocent game of strategy	140
NARCOTICS	**143**
PROVOCATIVE PSYCHOTHERAPY	**148**
A strike where it hurts	151

| Disorientation and relaxation | 159 |
| The approval | 160 |

| RELATIONS BETWEEN THE TWO SEXES | 164 |
| When biology is disregarded | 169 |

| DIVORCE: A WAR FOR FREEDOM | 178 |

PARENT – CHILD RELATIONSHIPS	184
Downgrading: A canker in a relationship	189
The contest of generations	191
The Rule of Three S	192

| TWO 'LOVING' SIBLINGS | 196 |

PEOPLE'S PERSONALITY	204
Hysterical personality	205
Compulsive personality	211

| THE DELAY IN PSYCHIATRY | 216 |

| WHAT HAS MEANING IN MY EXISTENCE? | 220 |

| SUICIDE | 223 |
| Why should I stay alive? | 229 |

THE PSYCHIATRIST'S MORAL DILEMMA	233
Antidepressants	233
Improvement with drops	236
Advice on eugenics	245

| PSYCHOANALYSIS: AN ATTEMPT TO CHANGE A BASIC PROGRAMME | 249 |

| IN LIEU OF AN AFTERWORD: PSYCHIATRY AND RATIONALISM | 253 |

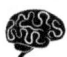

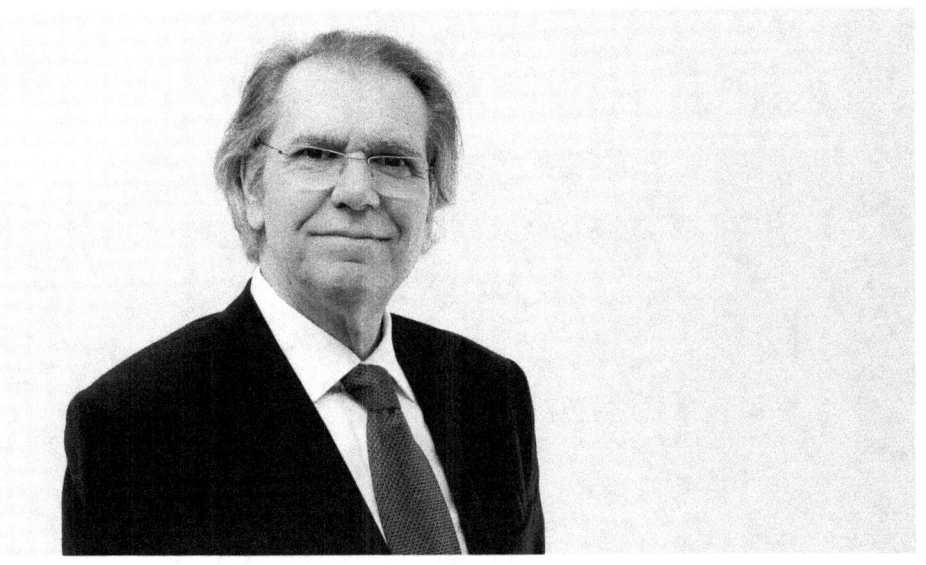

AUTHOR'S BIOGRAPHY

PAVLOS SAKKAS grew up in the milieu of psychiatry as his father was also a psychiatrist. Pavlos has practiced Psychiatry at the front line for the last thirty years and is a Professor of Psychiatry at the Medical School of the University of Athens. He has also been a Visiting Professor at the University of Illinois in Chicago. He has obtained prestigious scholarships and has accomplished substantial works in research, with hundreds of publications in international scientific journals.

However, despite these great professional achievements, his greatest fondness is for teaching. He has spent his long academic career initiating thousands of medical students and hundreds of specialised psychiatrists into the world of psychiatry. Furthermore, featuring in the media on numerous occasions, he tries to familiarise the general public with the messages of modern Psychiatry and the significant developments achieved in recent decades.

Pavlos Sakkas' inquisitive spirit has formulated fresh and enterprising points of view concerning certain aspects – that are still obscure – of psychiatry. In his clinical work, which has been met with high esteem, he has meanwhile applied special personal techniques of approach to a patient. It is these views and employed technique that are set out in his present book, which represents the distillation of his knowledge and experience.

A FEW WORDS ABOUT THE BOOK

THIS VOLUME contains the principal elements preoccupying modern Psychiatry. The author introduces the reader into all mental illnesses, on the one hand through real examples deriving from his rich clinical experience and on the other explaining in simple terms the 'fault' that is the underlying cause. It is in essence an interesting investigation into the magical world of the human brain. Using easily comprehended language, the author provides convincing explanations for the diverse mental functions. The models he expounds on bring mental illness down to earth from the mists of Philosophy to the realities of Medicine. He compares schizophrenia to a minor short–circuit, and Anorexia Nervosa to the activation of a programme in reserve in the brain. He gives reasons for the necessity for sleep and dreams.

Other than a doctor, however, Pavlos Sakkas is a person intensively querying social behaviour. His many years of practice of psychiatry and his experience of human pain give him the potential to be of assistance to those who arrive at crucial crossroads in their life. His charitable attitude and the unconventional viewpoints he develops provide interesting answers to the greatest existentialist questioning of human beings. He speaks of his own questioning and recounts what he answers when his patients ask him about the meaning of life.

In this book the reader will be able to find useful directions to be guided in the great and thrilling journey of life: Guidelines for relations with parents, siblings, companions and one's children.

The author has a way of transmitting such knowledge to his layman reader as would be envied by an experienced psychiatrist. But the book's best achievement is to bring the reader into the head and the thoughts of a psychiatrist. His way also at the same time gives advice in the correct practice of clinical Psychiatry as well as of Medicine in general.

It is a book addressing every challenged and questioning person who cogitates a problem, including professionals of mental health, who will find in it new methods of approach along the hazardous paths of the human soul.

INTRODUCTION

IN MY DAY, the school I went to was exceptional due to the in–depth Classical education it provided. I can still recall some philologists who were passionate about initiating us into the intellectual achievements of Ancient Greek philosophy and the emotions of the heroes of Greek tragedies.

I was immersed in this way not only in the nobility of Socrates' sacrifice for the ideals of justice, I also espoused the hallmark of Platonic philosophy, the famous 'know thy self'. And furthermore I was steeped in the Aristotelian view that Science sets out from formulation of the Why? Dialectics became the tool of my daily life and so I continue to this day to seek out alternative propositions which by juxtaposition will lead me nearer to 'The truth'.

Inevitably, therefore, I became a person governed by curiosity, who never accepts any received wisdom without trying to explain it, including myself and how I function. It was medicine that guided me to a constant quest – although the phrase may be expressed back to front – that is, that my need to explain everything that happens to me led me inevitably to medicine.

It is also evident that my choice to make my career in Academia as a university teacher and researcher is a sign of my obsessive search for knowledge. This was reinforced by my love of teaching, where on a daily basis I confront the querying of my students. Their queries are so often a trigger for a deeper delving into knowledge as well as to 'reread' familiar old postulations, seeing them from a fresh angle.

I confess, too, that I extend my position of a teacher who is willing to learn from his student to my relationship with my patients and their entourage. I always try to tell them everything they need to know about their illness, at the same time finding out about their own experience so as best to be able to help them.

To revert to my starting point, my school and my teachers acquainted me with the passions of the heroes of the Tragedies and their ineluctable destiny. I admit that the teenager that I was had admiration for the cleverness of Oedipus for solving the Riddle of the Sphinx, and his bravery for killing the king, but knowing as the reader that it was his father, I had doubts whether the act was heroic or criminal. We lived the emotions of the tragic protagonists intensely at my school and I too felt Electra's righteous fever, just as the compulsion of Orestes to see justice done.

My subsequent psychiatric studies later made me aware of the degree to which man is devoid of freedom in his development: I saw that in our life we resemble those heroes of ancient tragedy; we inescapably follow the route that has been laid down for us. We are simply executing the script of a scenario; it is exceedingly hard for us to overcome what we have been programmemed for.

This is the keyword that brought me to the writing of this book: all that I learned from psychiatry about the determining role that what we experience in early childhood plays in the decisions we make in the rest of our life may be compared to computer programming. Just as the computer cannot help but 'run' the programme loaded, a person cannot escape from what he or she has been 'taught' in the first years of life.

The word is in inverted commas because the first, decisive lessons of life are given without the slightest idea of the impact on the subsequent life of the infant. They are the earliest reactions of the person caring for the baby, to whom the crying is addressed. It is the lack of caring and the child's answer to this lack.

What's more, the repetition and the learning process per se, finally, and the reinforcement of the child's particular reaction depend on how successful the reply was to the child's requirement from the world that surrounds it. If, for instance, I learn that by insisting on my demand by continual crying I will be satisfied, I shall go on insisting for the rest of my life.

In fact I cannot control that particular model of reaction with my reasoning, when I see from the situations that this reaction of mine is not going to help me. Furthermore, I can't stop it even when I feel that my reaction could be harmful to me!

Of course, later in life we forge new programmes, for the new situations that confront us. We do however always build on the existing software, constantly forming new programmes, which in turn will also hem us in. We learn to smoke and then, although realising it destroys us we cannot rid ourselves of the habit.

To change a programme that has been loaded requires a great effort that can commence only following a severe shock. Reasoning and willpower are unfortunately not enough. What is vital is a major existentialist threat. A great fright that comes at us suddenly when it was not expected. This train of thought led me, step by step, to adopt an unusual manner of approach to my patients. It is what I later called 'a provocative psychotherapy'.

That is to say that, instead of agreeing with their viewpoint, the angle from which they see their problems – about which they are after all asking for my help – on the contrary I scold them for their decisions and give a fresh dimension to the analysis they make for me. I'm always looking for and bringing up the opposite views from those of my patients. I argue with them and show them that they are in that situation by their own choice, quite simply because they cannot get away from their foundational programmes, that is, the basis on which their view of the world.

As to the attempt to change that manner of confronting the problems, sadly, it is easily seen that there is absolutely no motivation to change anything at all. This seemingly accommodating way of staying on the familiar and beaten track is naught but the fear of the unknown that will come with any change.

Besides, all living organisms are conservative at heart. To be conservative is a fundamental element for the preservation of life. However, on the other hand, change and experimentation with something new – that which in a word is called 'innovation' is what leads to wondrous development.

Regarding the general comparison of the brain to a computer, it is what gave me the tools to fill in a number of gaps in my knowledge for my approach to mental sickness. The reader of this book will find in it some of the explanations I gave. They are the models that help, as much in comprehending mental symptoms – which for many people range from being incomprehensible to demonic – as in the grave mental disorders such as schizophrenia, depression, mania, anxiety, obsessive compulsive disorder and anorexia nervosa.

The book is addressed to all those who wish to find out something more about our brain function. It is couched in a new and original way, as I use it for my lectures to my students and residents in psychiatry. The comments received are usually positive, they are certainly beyond the boring academic 'tradition'. That is a word that contains also the notion of conservatism, something to which I am totally opposed, as the essence of my teaching is the spirit of querying all things.

I should finally like to let the reader know that examples of patients and interventions will be given in the various chapters. The examples are absolutely authentic but unavoidably, I had to omit and disguise any elements of identity from which the patient could be recognised. Patients might of course recognise their own case. This may bring back to mind situations that they want to forget, but they should think that the example helps others to understand the complex routes followed by the human brain.

I take this opportunity to thank all my patients, once again, for letting me learn from them and from my interaction with them. They have been my principal teachers and it is to them this book is dedicated.

A chapter about the history of Psychiatry explaining how contemporary psychiatric practice is directly related to psychopharmacology has been added to the second edition.

A chapter has also been added to the description of the function of the human brain that better helps us to understand how it works, especially the origins of the 'primitive' behaviors that have always affected the history of the human race. This analysis elucidates the direction in which these behaviors have been moving over time, as well as my own concerns, and hopefully, my future books.

Finally, I have added a new analysis to the chapter about human personalities, which is based on the subversive perspective that divides people into 'merchants' and 'scientists'.

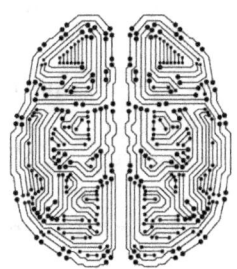

THE HUMAN BRAIN: AN ADMIRABLE COMPUTER

Memory

ON A BURNING hot noontime in Athens I was asked to do a medical examination of an elderly woman at her home in Kypseli, a middle–class, very lively urban neighborhood which is gradually being occupied by immigrants. The way there took me to a street where a girlfriend of mine once lived. In my younger days I often went there. For a long time that street was my beloved destination. I knew every inch of it. Going along it now, after such a long time, made me feel quite emotional.

The first thing that came into my mind was the fragrance of freshly baked bread from a bakery at the bottom of the street. I could smell a warm oven when my car windows were closed and the air conditioning was on! Obviously, the odour was 'saved' in my memory and now came up to my brain's 'desktop'.

No sooner had I though this than at the next corner I espied the door of a taverna where my girlfriend and I often ended up of an evening. It was a low door, and it was closed so that I had the fleeting impression the taverna must have closed down. Nevertheless, not only was I pervaded by the acidic smell of the barrels but I was reminded of the quarrelling of the owner with his wife which in the innocence of youth we found so amusing. Leaving the place, with our arms about one another we often wondered:

"What sort of marriage is that?" "How can they stand each other?" "When the fellow has been drinking he gets opinionated and abrupt, and she is a shrew who is always putting him down and scorning him". "She blames him for the failure of her dreams…"

Already then, when I was a young medical student, I tried to peek behind the surface and find the causes of words and actions. I tried not to fall into the facile position of the judge of actions and to be instead a judge of their causes, and especially, of intentions.

But out of all these reminiscences, I suddenly realised that lots of scenes were displayed on the 'screen' of my brain: videos with picture and sound as well as scents, tastes, contacts and, above all, sentiments. Millions of memory bytes, images my brain had been storing for decades. Memories that re–awakened with a wink from my mind as soon as I was in that particular street in a quarter of Athens.

And then I passed in front of the building where my first official love used to live. I nostalgically remembered the times we spent together in the flat when her parents were absent. And also, I remembered her friend and schoolmate who lived in the flat above. The girl's brother, the parents, and so much more…

It was but a spot on the map of Athens but it sprouted images and memories without end. It was as if I had hit a vein of artesian well water and it was pouring out under pressure. Liquid stored in a subterranean reservoir, years and years ago. This is how our brain is. It stores everything it perceives, with all its sensors, and it is ready to recall as soon as it is needed.

One little spot on the Athens town plan … A couple of blocks of a little street in Kypseli represented a huge quantity of memory stored in my brain. Then I caught sight of my car's GPS. It was a mechanism that I admired, until that moment. But, what does this extraordinary device tell me? Nothing but the name of the street. Meanwhile in my brain a million more pieces of data are stored for this particular street!

I bowed to my mind's superiority. From the time I was born, and maybe when I was still in the womb it must have been storing data. All the time. With the hours of sleep being the only time that the engine was ticking over in neutral. When asleep, the brain classifies the images it collected the foregoing day. For more than two thirds of our total lifetime during which we are awake (24 hours less 6 – 8 hours of sleep) we are recording what we see, what we hear, what we feel, with all our senses. It is quite possible in fact that we remember not only what we see with our central vision, that is what we look at, but also what is inscribed in our peripheral vision. So we do not only remember the figures and the places we observe but also those that go by without our noticing them.

And all these voluminous data always find free space to be stored. The most aged persons, 115 years old, have room in their brain that is free to store new information. Of course they have lost millions of neurons together with the information stored in them, but they have neurons with empty space to store new data!

It is natural for anyone with expertise in computers to feel awed before the capacity of memory of the human brain. In the minimal space lodged in our skull, all the data of our life can be stored. Everything we take in all the time through our senses as well as all we produce with our thought. We register pictures, sounds, tastes, odours, contacts, pain as well as joys and sadness, fears, ideas, viewpoints, even stories we made up, that is states and data we have manufactured with our creative thought.

An enormous quantity of data is constantly being imprinted on our brain, with unbelievable speed as well as with incredible stability that allows it to preserve them intact for many years. This is how years later we can still recall every detail of scenes we lived through or imagined.

Search engine

THE HUMAN brain is not only distinguished by its inexhaustible memory, it is also acts as an admirable search engine. For a brain to handle such an enormous volume of data, it first needs to have an equally powerful search mechanism. And our brain has the best of them.

I went to the police station recently to renew my passport and was asked to provide a photograph 'with special specifications' for my face to be recorded in the international files. Modern technology requires the face to be expressionless and facing the lens. That is the only way what I look like can be differentiated among the millions of photographs in the files.

I can't forget the day when, many years ago, I went to New York for the first time and was walking along Fifth Avenue. Amongst the crowd of people from the four corners of the earth hurrying on their way, on the opposite pavement I caught sight of Sophia, a cousin of mine. I didn't know she was also in New York and for a moment I hesitated. Anyway I couldn't see her clearly as she was ahead of me and on the other side of the road. But I could tell from how she moved, looking into shop windows, from her clothes, her hair, that it was Sophia. I walked faster, crossed over and sure enough, it was she! We were both astounded. How could I have recognised her, in amongst such a crowd, and without looking for her either! It is evident my brain's search engine is working all the time and is constantly ceaselessly making thousands of cross–references.

For this extraordinary feat to be realised, a subtracting capability is necessary as well as a capacity for synthesis. The processor can on the one hand pinpoint the typical facets of a subject, a representation, so as to be able to pick it out only by means of them. On the other hand, recognising only one or two typical points, the whole representation can be put together.

The cleverness is not in the memorisation of the elements but in their classification and the capacity to seek out that element that is required at any moment. This is how we can compare elements and draw conclusions, what we call judgment: Which is the best route or even who is the best companion (the supreme quest for most people)?

In the extraction of these conclusions we are assisted by the search engine we have in our brain. This will help us retrieve those elements from our memory for the case of each route so as to be able to compare them. In fact, in seeking out the elements of alternative routes, corresponding search filters are necessary so as to exclude information irrelevant to the initial question. If what is sought is the quickest route, the filters will omit details of buildings or the parks or flower–beds on another route. But if the prettiest scenic route is what is wanted, the filters will focus on those beautifying aspects and omit the details of traffic and waiting at traffic lights.

It is the search engine that makes humans rational beings but its effectiveness is due to language, the voiced representation of data. Language, initially only spoken and then written, enabled the grouping of things and notions. This then enabled the capacity to abstract and the formation of notions and things.

I do not know if my computer will one day be able to communicate with me elliptically and abstractedly, leaving out the self–evident. I doubt it though. Until then, the human brain will be the most perfect mechanism on the earth.

Plasticity: a gift as well as a jail

WHEN I WAS a medical student, in Physiology the current view was that the human brain was composed of a multitude of neural networks which had a given interconnection. In fact, our professor used to show us a print–out of some transistor radio network and told us that millions of such networks consisting of neural cells with their nerve–ends controlled the brain's function. This was in the 70s, when printed networks signified evolution in applied technology.

However, in the next decade it appeared that the networks and interconnections of our brain are not fixed, nor are they rigid. Neurons, that are nerve–cells, have a particularity called plasticity. They are able to modify their interconnections, their 'branches' one could say, with which they communicate with their neighboring neurons. You can visualise it as two trees next to one another, which, if needed, can develop branches from one to the other so as to be able to communicate.

In the case of the neurons, the communication of one 'branch' with that of a neuron close by takes place by a chemical process, with substances we call neurotransmitters, such as acetylcholine, noradrenaline, serotonin, dopamine and others. If one branch emits dopamine for instance, it can communicate only with other branches that can be stimulated by dopamine, meaning they have dopamine receptors. This is how selective stimulation is achieved, between 'branches' speaking the same language. In this way, communication is not diffused but instead is directed along specific 'paths'.

Recent discoveries have revealed that what we call the brain's plasticity has an energy enabling certain 'branches' to change language if necessary when communicating with other 'branches' around them, thus creating new communication networks. If, for example, a neuron produced serotonin with one of its 'branches' and could communicate with neighbouring 'branches' having serotonin receptors, this 'branch' can, if necessary, 'learn' to produce dopamine, so as to be able to communicate with another 'branch' that has dopamine receptors.

The discovery of the brain's nerve–cell plasticity altered the theories we had about our brain's function. Nowadays we believe that the brain is a 'living' computer. It has the capacity to be transformed according to its function and its needs. It has the capacity to change the interconnections among its neurons, to open contacts and create fresh networks. It seems to have the potential to create far more interconnections than it employs in practice.

Our brain resembles a fallow field in which many paths may be opened according to the direction in which we guide our thoughts and how we act. The more often we use a path, the better it is freed and thus becomes negotiable and ready to use.

In fact, the administration of our brain's economy makes us employ the easiest paths, the most practicable. Only if our brain is required to operate a new function does the bulldozer come into play to open a new path, a new route of contact among the 'branches' of specific neurons requisite for that particular function to be feasible.

The capacity to open new paths and routes is our brain's great strength. It is as if it had 'shortcuts' to facilitate the operation of our computers; speedy networks to give us easy access to what we want to be activated.

We all remember what an effort it took for the first ten kilometres when we started driving. Our brain was continuously trying to coordinate our feet on the pedals, our hands on the wheel and gears and our eyes to the front and to the mirrors. After a few miles, however, our movements were more easily coordinated and after a few days we drove almost automatically, without thinking or trying to calculate our every move.

Our brain has a wonderful particularity of effortlessly creating automatic conditions. It is its way of operating efficiently.

We can therefore easily understand that our brain's plasticity – that is its capacity to process programmes for the execution of all the operations concerning it – is responsible for all that constitutes what we call 'human civilization'.

Habit: a gift to burn your fingers

THIS ADMIRABLE characteristic function of our brain to take shortcuts, to automate, is what leads us to what we call habits. There are good ones and others not so good or even bad. Habits economise the work our brain has to do but at the same time lays traps for it. It traps us into relying on programmes we no longer have any use for. We learned to read and no longer spell "b a ba" as we did, but on the other hand we also learned to eat sweets, to smoke and to be couch potatoes in front of the TV.

But unfortunately, or fortunately for us, once the human brain installs a shortcut it cannot be uninstalled. In that, it is not like our computers, where we can uninstall a shortcut. In a human being it is instead like the saying, 'You never forget how to ride a bike'. It means that years later, automatic balance and operation of the pedals are there, ever present to be used if needed.

This is what I call the jail of our destiny because when we face a particular query, the answer does not come freely but depends on our past and the previous answers we gave to this particular question. The routes we followed in the past are the easiest ones and the answers thus spring forth without us thinking about them or questioning them. The ready–made shortcuts come into operation because that is in the best interest of our brain. We are condemned to give the same answer, the one we elaborated before when the question was the same. So, irrespective of the present phase, where circumstances have changed and our mature thought indicates a different direction, our immediate response that springs to mind will nevertheless be the one used before.

The totality of these shortcuts, or automatic responses, constitutes what we call a person's character or personality. They are the prompt answers everyone gives to basic questions.

Obviously, these life attitudes were in essence learned in the first years of life and are subsequently repeated, almost automatically. For reasons of economy, the brain doesn't take the trouble to reconfirm whether the programmes it is using already configured are the right ones. You could say the person has blind confidence in the programmes that they themselves downloaded in the past.

The Hardware and Software in Our Brains

IN SUMMARY, one can think of our brain as a wonderful computer that on the one hand has a number of inbuilt programs with which we were born, and on the other, programs it has acquired over the course of its life. The basic programs we inherited from our biological ancestors form a kind of hardware, in computer terms, which is already running in our brains at birth.

These hardware programs control our essential bodily functions such as respiration, heart, and digestion. However, this hardware also includes programs that compel us to seek food, and to protect ourselves from adverse environmental conditions, as well as from our enemies. In other words, these programs ensure our personal survival.

Finally, our hardware also regulates our reproductive programs in order to safeguard the survival of the species. Since sexual arousal is in our genome, it is already installed in our brain and does not need to be learned. This is why we often see children exhibit sexual stimulation before they are able to understand the true purpose of this pleasant sensation. Because the socio-ethical norms of today demand that the operation of this program is 'paused', or put into the 'freezer', extra software programs to obstruct the source of sexual stimulation are manufactured immediately. Unfortunately some of these inhibitory programs can adversely affect future spontaneous sexual function and lead to sexual dysfunction after adolescence.

All human brains contain programs similar to those that determine the survival behaviors of most animals as individuals and as a species. Modern civilized man tends to shun these programs because they involve many 'primitive' behaviors that are now considered either obsolete or contrary to the moral codes formulated over the 15,000 years we have lived in organized societies. However, since there is no method to 'uninstall' these programs they can never be completely erased.

Nevertheless, it is important that we recognize that our brains contain programs that, for example, foster greed, opportunism, and arrogance. We see this also in animal behaviors where the strongest beast claims the 'lion's share', disregarding the needs of its fellows in favour of its own personal survival. Such behaviors may be inhibited in most people, but they can arise under the right circumstances. It is not surprising, therefore, that whoever is in a position of power may take it for granted that they are entitled to more benefits, and greater latitude within the law. Ethics and education can limit these 'primitive' behaviors, but we must accept that the beast is always within us.

A study of the history of the human race shows that it is precisely these programs that have led all our endeavors for social equality to ruin. It was the 'primitive' nature of the human brain that undermined the French Revolution, when warring leaders slaughtered each other in their battle for supremacy. Indeed the neglect of these 'primitive' instincts by the theorists of social ideology resulted in the derailment of the socialist experiments of the C20th. The pursuit of individual gain is not an abstract model of the theory of capitalism, but a pre-installed program in the brains of every human being.

Another example of our inherited programs is our innate tendency to ignore the trap and grab the 'cheese'. We cannot resist the temptation presented by easy gain, and constantly find that logic is powerless to contain our impulse to take the bait. Populist politicians exploit this by making promises that are irresistible to those who are unwilling to heed the logic and the warnings of the wise.

Education and moral codes are able only to limit the occasional greed we all tend to manifest. No law however, has the power to abolish these programs since they are embedded in the human brain.

On the other hand, herd animals have a pre-installed program that favors mutual support within the group. For example when a single buffalo is attacked, the rest of the herd unites to protect it, and then fight back. Most herd animals manifest these behaviors because their inherited programs promote solidarity. Solidarity is fundamental to our philanthropic activities, since philanthropy is both a cultivated behavior, and an instinct based on the needs of the group.

So why after so many millennia, is mankind yet to create a world of peace and prosperity? The answer lies in the fact that the expression of programs concerning individual survival takes precedence over those concerned with the survival of the group. Only the sated beast will permit its fellows to approach its food.

The hardware we have inherited from our ancestors determines our behavior. No matter how much he may want to, man cannot escape the biology that defines him as Homo sapiens.

Our software consists of programs installed in our brains post birth. The earliest of these are a result of imitation when a newborn watches and attempts to copy movements, sounds and facial expressions. Later software depends less on mimicry and more on conscious learning, for example, a baby very soon learns that crying results in receiving attention and the feeling of being loved. Once these behaviors are consolidated with frequent rewards, they become foundational to our personality and character.

Our software includes tiny, complex programs, along with shortcuts and other connections that are a result of repeated attempts and reiterations. Talking, walking, ball play, swimming, cycling, and horse riding, are just a few of the programs we have installed through imitation, learning, exercise, and continual practice, to develop an easier and more economical performance of the brain. Programs that we established from early childhood are the result of our own efforts, with perhaps some general instructions. They can, for example, manifest as courtesy, meanness, courage, or sociability.

Unfortunately, or fortunately, there are no ready-made apps such as those developed for mobile phones, for our brains. Combined with the influence of our parents, teachers and friends, and our personal experiences, we create all our own software. Indeed the stories we have heard from others, even if they are distortions or fantasies, are easily imported into our own experiences.

Fairy tales, novels, television, cinema, and social media, produce a counterfeit reality that our brain inadvertently incorporates into its own authentic reality experiences. This constantly evolving patchwork is the basis upon which our mind forms its conclusions and responses to the myriad of stimuli it receives daily.

The extent to which the bogus reality influences our ideology is often absurdly apparent in televised interviews when bemused witnesses claim to be 'flabbergasted' by the arrest of a neighbor they never suspected to be 'bad'. Cinema and television have 'taught' us that the 'bad guys' are ugly, secretive, badly groomed and wear dark colours. Casting demands that only the good have angelic faces. Thus the software that guides us in our decision-making often turns out to be wrong because is it based on cliché.

The sham reality that has flooded our lives has filled our minds with misinformation, and the only tool we have to filter it out is critical thinking. Modern man must exercise his judgment in order to reject those scenarios that manipulate his behavior against his own interests. The less we consume this pre-digested intellectual fare, and the more we seek out truth, the more our lives will be governed by our own authentic goals and aspirations and not by the values imposed on us by others.

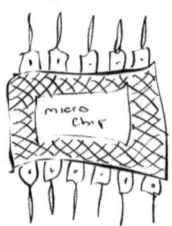

SCHIZOPHRENIA: A TINY SHORT-CIRCUIT

I WAS in my office at the hospital one spring morning when, after knocking at the door, a lady of about fifty years old came in. She was wearing a white hospital gown.

— *May I come in?*

— *Please do, take a seat.*

— *I'm a pharmacist at the hospital next door, and I would like your advice about my son.*

— *What's the matter with your son?*

— *My boy was top of his class at school and one of the first in university entrance exams.*

I may sound like a bit of a cynic but I have learned from experience that when a mother begins a description of her son in this way, it will be a case of schizophrenia. The overwhelming majority of parents with children who suffer from schizophrenia tend to embellish the behaviour and the achievements of the offspring before the illness was manifested. I think they do this for two reasons:

Firstly it is to cover up some hereditary trait in their family. Something hereditary the entire family keeps under seal in the greatest secrecy. The naïve reasoning they project even to themselves is that since the child was normal until the age of 18, the condition cannot be due to genes that could have been handed down from so–and–so, the uncle who is 'nervy' and had spent time in a psychiatric clinic. The parents think: "if my child had some hereditary defect, it would have appeared at birth." Unfortunately this is completely wrong; a number of hereditary disturbances, such as baldness for example, appear much later in a person's life.

A second reason for embellishing the sufferer's behaviour in childhood is to refute the guilt that parents nearly always feel about the upbringing of their sick child. You see, psychiatry has done a good job! And indeed, it is generally believed in society that schizophrenia may be due to a lack of love or early abuse, physical or mental, of a child. Consequently, as soon as the parents realise that there is something seriously wrong with their child, they try either to deny it by shutting it out of their mind by pretending they don't see it, or they protest that they gave their child the best upbringing they could. If they have more than one child, straight away they will tell – themselves as well as others – that all their children were brought up the same way: *"I never made any difference between them, Doctor."*

– *"… He must have had an unhappy love affair at university and he has been depressed ever since. He shut himself away into himself, he isolated himself, he wouldn't go to lectures and eventually quit his studies …"*

Classically, parents will try to put the blame of their child's disease onto some third person. Very often, as in this case, some girl who broke up with their boy. Of course if one investigates it will appear that the girl realised the young man had a problem and kept her distance. But, for most parents it was her fault because it was when she left him that he became ill.

Another approach – that I would call classic – is that the early symptoms of schizophrenia are seen as depression. It is often the sense of being threatened from the environment that the schizophrenic feels that makes them withdraw into isolation. They may shut themselves indoors or into their room, close doors and windows and draw the curtains so as not to be seen from the outside – by those they think are watching – and won't go out. Such refuge in isolation and darkness is therefore easily seen as symptoms of depression. It is made worse by the fact that very often the sufferers will not talk about it (because they think others are listening). This is also why some patients speak in a very low voice. In some cases in fact, in the early stages some schizophrenics lose weight, not from anorexia as happens in depression, but because they are afraid of being poisoned. It may therefore happen that a doctor, seeing the symptoms only, may be misled into thinking that the isolation, the lack of incentive to do anything, the weight loss, are all due to depression.

– *How old is your son?*

— *He's 28. But since he was 22 he has in effect given up any effort to pass any tests at his college and has shut himself away into himself, he started occupying himself with the Church. He only left the house to go to church. He read religious books, fasted and prayed.*

— *Does he talk to himself?*

— *He prays aloud, he's often mumbling, and recently he seems to be talking to Jesus Christ. His room is full of icons and he burns incense.*

— *Why did you wait so long to see a psychiatrist?*

I have to admit that I have sometimes been known to be abrupt with parents. It's because I know that delaying therapy increases the damage to the patient's brain and makes therapy more difficult. Of course as a psychiatrist, I understand how hard it is for a parent to face the fact that his or her child has a severe and chronic illness. That is just why they are prepared to believe that it is the 'evil eye' or a curse. There are instances where they think the change in behaviour is because the child was taken by the Church and fell under its influence, or that it is due to political convictions. It seems that for a parent anything is preferable to facing the fact that the child may have a mental illness, namely schizophrenia.

— *Like I said, at first we thought the melancholy from the unhappy love affair would pass. We encouraged him to go out, to meet another girl. But, as he wasn't going to college, he got cut off. His grandmother took him to a priest for a blessing to see if that would comfort him, and ever since he has turned to the Church… His relation to the Church has become closer and closer, but he went to church less often. He transformed his room into a church. He told us he wanted to become a monk. We did everything to dissuade him… Doctor, did we do something wrong?*

— *Well, even if he had gone to a monastery, he would still have been ill. The illness is inside him. Wherever he goes, he will carry it in his brain.*

I try to give the biological dimension of schizophrenia as early as possible in my diagnosis. It relieves the parents from their guilt. I want to transmit the message that their child's sickness is just like all the other physical illnesses. Would they feel guilty if the child was short-sighted, or had asthma or diabetes? In the same way they should not feel guilty about a mental disorder.

— *Do you think it wasn't the disappointment in love, Doctor?*

— *Lots of people fall in love and it's rejected. God help us if they all became ill as your son did. His trouble was neither the unhappy love affair nor your behaviour. It isn't a question of upbringing. Circumstances are probably just the trigger. The cause was in his brain from birth. He had the predisposition and as soon as he was under pressure the problem emerged.*

— *You mean he would have fallen ill anyway?*

— *This is what we believe nowadays. And if he hadn't fallen ill because of that incident, it would have happened later, let's say when he did his military service. But tell me, what state is he in now?*

— He's shut in his room and comes out only to eat and go to the bathroom. He burns incense and prays...

— Or, he's talking to God.

— Maybe. He sometimes gives the impression he's talking to saints. Then at other times he's in his own world, he seems to be looking but he isn't seeing...

It is heartrending to see parents who are certainly aware that there's something wrong with their child but will yet not admit that it is an illness. They try to explain away their bizarre behaviour and so do not get medical help early enough. And this mother is a pharmacist – from the sphere of medicine! Even so, her son's state had to reach the limit for her to seek assistance from a doctor. It was easier for her to take him to a spiritual adviser. Because, inevitably, seeing a doctor would mark him as 'mad', what parents will not come to terms with in any way as if it was the label that's the problem and not the illness itself, which has a name, understandably painful. But, unfortunately, avoiding the labeling does not avoid the problem.

In just the same way there are people who realise that they have cancer but won't go to the doctor. Some time ago, when I was at the General Hospital, there was a woman who came to see the gynecologist only when her breast was bleeding so much she could no longer hide it from her husband. She had cancer, of course, at an advanced stage and she had obviously known it – her mother and her sister had both died of breast cancer. But so as to gain a little time of mental peace, she had preferred to hide it from her family, even from her own self!

— And what does your son do all day?

— He lies on his bed. He gets up to go to the toilet. He hasn't washed for a month and now that it's Lent he hasn't eaten for a week. He just drinks water. That too, he gets it himself from the tap and drinks it only when he has said a 'prayer' over it, as he says.

— You tell me, what can I do about this?

This is a question I always ask to find out how they expect me to intervene. The intervention might seem evident in this case, but it isn't always so. A doctor shouldn't pre–empt the patient or the relative. It very often happens that they expect the doctor to reassure them that there's nothing wrong or that they need not do anything as things will get better on their own, in time.

I have heard all sorts of suggestions: "Don't you think, Doctor, <u>we</u> should talk about this?" "Perhaps he ought to have sex?" They sound most peculiar to me – I might say, tragic, but for those desperate people they are a ray of hope.

– *You know, Doctor, I'm afraid he's going to die of starvation. He has to be hospitalised, right away. As a colleague from the nearby hospital, I'm asking you to admit him to your unit – I've heard it's one of the best.*

– *Thank you very much. We do try to do our best.*

Flattery is something a doctor needs immunisation to. He has to show he is flattered, because if he doesn't, it makes him appear superior, not taking the bait, and his interlocutor will feel rejected; but at the same time not let the flattery enter past the surface of his mind. It is, you see, a matter of delicate balance.

– *I shouldn't think your son will like to be taken to hospital. He won't admit to being ill…*

Of course I wanted to add that "when you yourself won't admit he's ill, do you expect him to do so?" But that would have been too much for her, and I restrained myself.

– *His father and I have agreed to tell him to come to the hospital chapel for the service of its saint's day in two days' time, and you will then take him in.*

– *Madam, we aren't dog–catchers taking strays off the streets. Even if we could bring him in here, we can't hold anyone against their will. The only way to hospitalise someone forcibly is through the legitimate procedure of the public prosecutor's warrant. You have to go to the prosecutor and asked to have your son examined by two psychiatrists. The prosecutor will issue an order to your area police to send someone to your address, to take the patient away for examination. If the psychiatrists determine that your son is ill and refuses therapy he needs, they will then certify to the prosecutor that he must be forcibly hospitalised. The prosecutor will order the procedure to be carried out, and then we can admit him and put him through the treatment he needs. Consequently, the first thing you have to do is go to the public prosecutor. This is the legal procedure in our country.*

As a process, this may seem inhuman, or violent, or bureaucratic, but it is nevertheless the optimum balance between individual rights and the right to treatment. I remember that in Chicago, for someone to be hospitalised against their will they had to proclaim before a judge that they wanted to kill somebody or themselves. The judge would come to the clinic and ask the patient if he or she wanted to kill someone. If the patient denied it the judge would order the clinic to let him go, even if it was obvious the patient was talking to himself and was severely ill. This was supposed to serve 'the liberty of the individual'. What of course was served was the taxpayers' money because if the patient was not subjected to obligatory treatment he or she would usually be made a homeless person and in the winter would die of cold – the minus 20 or 30 degrees in the winter, of Chicago, New York, Detroit, Washington DC and most cities of North America.

When I talked to my American colleagues about this social injustice, which is what this behaviour toward schizophrenics seems to me to be, as well as to politicians in the States, I was astounded by the cynicism of most of them. They would initially advance arguments in favour of freedom of the individual and his wish to live as he wanted to, on condition that he did no harm, of course. "Since he isn't going to kill anyone, let him live the way he wants."

I would then tell them that a schizophrenic's judgment is influenced by the confusion reigning in their brain and that consequently it is not a case of free choice. In fact I insisted that what they were saying about the 'freedom' as like letting a blind person to be free to choose where to go. "Whether left or right, sooner or later they would be destroyed. They must first of all have their vision repaired if we can, and then let them go out to be free to choose." That was when I would hear, from most of them, that most cynical reply: "And why should I, an American taxpayer, pay for the blind man's cure?"

To close this chapter I wish to declare that in view of the foregoing I am totally unmoved by the surprise and the mourning of society following every 'inexplicable' massacre in schools, colleges and mass gatherings of people. Those are crocodile tears shed to cover what is in essence the indifference of society toward the disabled. Not to speak of the fact that the freedom to bear arms – valid in most States – makes criminals of many schizophrenics. The unhappily sick people who, in a delirium of their condition, may be screaming or fighting with some unsuspecting and unknowing opponent, who they think is stalking them or going to murder them, or were sent by the Devil to tempt them. If they have a gun in their pocket, these strange or grotesque 'madmen' become criminals.

Now this particular young man, as his mother told me, heard Jesus Christ speak to him and give him instructions. Because he was a mild person himself, so far he had not expressed any tendency to aggression. He was just trying to defend himself against the aggression he felt from others. Of course, nobody can ever know to what degree the sufferer can feel pressurised or at a dead end and fall into despair. He may then suddenly become aggressive or he may commit suicide, a leap toward 'liberty'.

This is why the aggressiveness of schizophrenics appears unprovoked and inexplicable. They may think all at once that the person opposite is saying things against them and be therefore convinced that that person belongs to the gang who is stalking them and may feel they have no way out, and if they have a way – that is to say a weapon – they might cause 'unprovoked' harm.

When the next day the procedure with the prosecutor had been followed, the pharmacist's son, his name is Costas, was brought to the hospital by two police officers. He looked like something out of a Byzantine icon: long hair and beard, emaciated face, sunken cheeks, large and prominent eyes. Despite the distress he will certainly have felt at being removed from his surroundings by two strangers, he had the aspect of the martyr who does not resist the torments to which 'the enemies of his faith' were subjecting him. His expression was serene, springing from his compassion.

I introduced myself as well as the colleagues sitting in my office, a young psychiatrist, two psychiatric residents and two medical students. I have a teaching post at the hospital as well as practice as clinician. What I hope to do is transmit my knowledge, but especially my stance as a doctor, to my students and the residents in psychiatry. This is why I always examine my patients in the presence of my students.

The first time I saw this manner of examination was when I was a student myself, and I thought it must be very uncomfortable for the patient. To be examined in front of a lot of people is not conducive to opening one's soul. But, believe me, I manage to have a satisfactory emotional contact with all my patients, irrespective of how many people are there. I think it is an absolutely subjective matter to be capable of opening up and make a basic contact of sentiments. It could be in a crowded stadium. What counts is how the doctor will treat the case at hand. If the impression of an interrogation is given, it's to be expected that a patient will be on the defensive and not open up. If on the other hand they see a person opposite who sincerely wants to be of help, they will not only unburden their heart, they will also stretch out a hand to ask for help.

The young man cast an exploratory glance around the office and over the people sitting in it. Then his look stopped at me. The park and the Athens hill of Lycabettus could be seen from the window behind me, so I don't know if he was admiring the view or gazing at me, or even if he was considering an escape route from the window. It's natural that, at the start, patients admitted to hospital against their will feel they are imprisoned and look for a way out.

When a few hours or days later they comprehend the nursing routine of the psychiatric clinic, they accept that they have to stay there and at the same time also resign themselves to their medication treatment, since they realise right away that it is unavoidable. Usually, if a patient will not take the pills, the medication is administered by injection.

Even the most disturbed patient has the capacity of understanding 'where the wind is blowing from' and what can be done to bargain. Therefore, it is up to the nursing team to transmit a clear message that certain things are non–negotiable. Some of these are taking the medication and the obligation for all to follow rules of good behaviour. There can be no screaming, nor disturbing of the others, patients or staff. Nor can they demand special treatment such as they probably get at home from their family.

If on the other hand the patients understand that we are truly trying to help, then they all respond and cooperate with the doctors and nurses. The intention of doctors and staff needs only to be genuine because, however disturbed patients may be, they can tell when an effort is sincere and what the people around really feel. Communicating sentiments is, besides, the first thing a being develops at birth. Speech and spoken communication is a wonderful human creation which however can not only distort information, it can at times also spoil it and transmit erroneous messages. Sentiment on the contrary, that is the 'communication of the heart', as the poet says, never lies.

The look in Costas' eyes, although searching, nevertheless had a serenity found in profoundly religious persons. He was looking at us not as a hunted wild animal but as testifying to his faith to those who threw him into the arena with the beasts.

– *Costas, your mother told us you aren't eating properly lately. And you do look very thin. She worries, quite rightly, about your health, and that's why you are here with us. We want you to eat normally so that there's no danger to your life. As you understand, it is we who are now responsible for your good health. If you don't like some of the food at the clinic, tell us and we'll find an alternative solution.*

– *My mother needn't have worried. I am fasting, and God is always with me and protecting me. No one has any reason to worry about me. I am in the hands of God. His Providence is great.*

– *That is the truth, but if something happens to you here in the clinic, human law will ask us what happened. And you must realise that no judge will accept that Divine Providence looked after you… Simply, we will go to jail because of you although it isn't our fault. Therefore I have to tell you I have no intention of going to prison and not being with my family just because you want to fast. As you believe in God, Costas, I'm sure you know He would not want this. You can communicate with God and take part in the divine without harming your fellows.*

A psychiatrist has to be quick–witted and have arguments ready to support his views. The major part of his work is playing ping–pong with his patients and their relatives. He has to be quick on the uptake and find answers that get him out of the impasse of the patient's logic. Inventiveness of arguments is a great advantage for a psychiatrist. Usually I go with the patient's logic and follow it, but I go beyond it, farther than they do. I surpass the patient's limits, and frequently, from the other side it can be seen that the patient's reasoning is overturned. The truth of every argument can be turned on its head if you stretch it out beyond 'common' logic. Isn't common logic what generally entraps us in conservative positions? If we supersede it, it guides us to unexpected results.

– *I have no intention of harming anyone. All I want is to purify my soul from the burden of my unclean body.*

– *Costas, I think you can find ways of purification without doing any harm, unwittingly, of course, to some fellow beings.*

I stressed the word 'unwittingly', so as to show him I was on his side. One must on no account go over to the other side. There are two things I avoid at any cost: to dispute my interlocutors and to put them on the defensive. If they are on the defensive they have to put up fortifications to hide behind, whereas what is required is for them to open up and trust you. Do not forget, the ultimate goal is to gain the confidence of the interlocutor.

— *I have begun a fast, alone in my room. My action is nobody's business but my own.*

— *Obviously, God directed you.*

— ...

— *Each of us has a way of communicating with God and finding a direction, especially when we are at a crossroads in our life.*

— *Are you a believer, Doctor?*

— *Everybody has faith ...*

I showed him, with a look in its direction, the icon I have in my office. A psychiatrist should always have some religious symbol in the office. Most patients either have some 'involvement' with religion, or simply place their hopes on it. Therefore they wish the psychiatrist to be on the same side as they. If on the contrary they gather that the psychiatrist is ideologically opposed to them, it is to be expected they will take up a defensive position, which is disastrous for a doctor–patient relationship as well as in general for the therapeutic alliance.

— *You know, Costas, it's simply that some people don't want to admit to it.*

— *So, Doctor, as you're a believer, you have to let me go on the road I have chosen.*

— *But what if in my opinion it is the road to perdition? Then, as a good Christian it's my obligation to prevent you and save you.*

— *Look here, Doctor, I shall accept to leave the road I have taken, solely so as not to involve you in my actions. I don't want you involved in any way because of my actions. But that doesn't mean I give up on my decisions.*

— *Of course, the decision is always yours to make. And in the Future you will be able to do whatever you wish. But for now you must allow me not to be involved in any way and I shall now proceed to fulfil my moral duty ...*

It often happens, even in cases of the most paranoid and aggressive patient, that once they are in the clinic, they realise they will not get their own way and will seek some excuse to retreat from the positions that – outside the clinic – they stated were non–negotiable. Consequently, the psychiatrist has to provide the patient with some excuses for an honorable retreat, without transmitting a message that it is a defeat. The polar positions of winner and loser have to be avoided at all costs. The doctor must have in mind above all things to establish a therapeutic alliance.

— I want to come back to my initial question, Costas: does God speak to you directly or does He send you His commandments through the intermediary of a saint?

— Through Saint Anthony.

— The rich man of the desert. The one who gave away his possessions after listening to the Gospel and became a hermit in the desert for years. All he ate was bread that was brought to him every six months. Wasn't it he who consolidated monasticism?

— Yes, exactly. That's why he instructed me to take the path of abstinence.

General knowledge always helps to get close to the interlocutor. It facilitates the effort to gain their confidence and to give them the feeling that they are understood. Contrariwise, for me my patients are an inexhaustible source of knowledge. While examining them I consciously interrupt the medical history with questions about the region they come from, their professional occupation, even their views on various topics. As a tactic, besides the opportunity it gives me to acquire amazing information, it breaks the ice, makes the other proud of his origins, his job, his knowledge.

Never shall I forget a lady I was once examining in the presence of a colleague. At some point she asked me what my sign of the zodiac was. Not only did I tell her, I even challenged her to guess my planetary ruler. My colleague, who knows my absolutely rational views on and my scorn for astrology could not help smiling. In fact when in the next question I mentioned the position of Venus in my astral chart, he couldn't restrain his laughter and had to rush out of the office with his hand over his mouth. Nevertheless, because of my knowledge of the subject I had won over the particular patient and had made a powerful therapeutic bond with her!

— And I suppose, Costas, the saint talks to you all the time and tells you what to do.

— He always tells me what to do so that I can achieve the heavens.

He had softened. At last he had found someone who understood him and didn't put him right or try to prove him wrong. Schizophrenics do not reveal their delusions, because they know everyone they tell will say that it isn't so and that it is all a figment of their imagination. If they had ever dared to tell the people close to them, those will have scolded the patient or, at best, assured them that it isn't possible. So it is natural that if they find someone who accepts these illusions as really existing phenomena, they feel they are believed and are comfortable in their communication with them.

A psychiatrist therefore has to accept the sick person's illusory experience, sincerely, just as the general practitioner accepts the subjective symptoms his patient recounts. There is no point in trying to convince the patient that his delusions are not real. It is like trying to convince someone who says he has toothache that it doesn't hurt or that the pain is much less than what the person says it is. If on the contrary they see their grievances taken into account, they will come to trust us. However, on no account may the psychiatrist confirm the delusions, telling the patient that he too hears the voice of Saint Anthony, nor can he accept the paranoiac's fantasy that the CIA is after him or that his wife has a lover. In such cases it is recommended to take the position of "if you say so, I accept it, although I think it is very improbable." It means we must not align ourselves with the delusion, while accepting it, keeping our stringent reservations and critical stance as to its existence. But not rejecting it.

– *Tell me, Costas, does the voice of St Anthony sound familiar?*

– *At first I thought it was one of my college teachers, but later I could tell it was the Saint.*

– *Weren't you scared the first time you heard it?*

– *Oh yes, in fact I tried to avoid it in every way. That's why I didn't go to classes and stayed at home.*

– *But then you heard it at home.*

– *I thought it came from the flat next door.*

– *Did it threaten you? Was that why you didn't want to hear it?*

– *Yes it did. It said I was a nothing, not worth anything. It was like being persecuted.*

– *Did you ever hear it from the TV?*

– *I did. How did you know that, doctor? There were times when on the television they were talking about me.*

– *Not openly, I think. They were insinuating things.*

– *Yes, oh yes. Usually, in the news. They would say something about me or they talked about my girlfriend. That's why I broke up with her. But it was no use ... They said negative things about me and my relationship with her. That's when I began sensing the presence of St Anthony. He said, quite calmly, that I mustn't worry about the comments of evil people, just that I must avoid them.*

– *So you stopped watching television.*

– *It's an instrument of Satan.*

– *You may be right.*

I said it with a smile, to lighten the atmosphere, which it did, confirmed by all those present. Costas looked at them enquiringly, perhaps slightly suspiciously, in case they were mocking him, but I had won him over. He knew I was dealing with him honestly and with sincerity. One could tell he really needed to talk – to someone, of course, who took him seriously and did not contest him.

— Ever since, I shut myself up into my room. I was concentrating and taking instructions from St Anthony.

— How did you know it was the saint?

— That's right, I didn't at the start. In fact I thought it was God.

— But?

— One day, when I had started abstinence, the saint revealed himself. That's how I was guided to fasting, absolute isolation and constant prayer.

— The course you took is perfectly understandable. But I don't know where it might lead you. While you are here with us, we will not press you to give up your isolation except for what is absolutely necessary. There is an isolation room where you will be by yourself. You can eat there, alone. But what we want from you is that you take your medication without fail and eat at least the minimum to stay alive.

Nothing is served by waging useless battles and opening up fronts when it can be avoided. The priority for a patient with schizophrenia is that they should take their medication. If the treatment is properly administered they will soon be more cooperative and we shall be able to put them within the desired bounds.

— Doctor, I don't need medication. What I need is His saving grace.

— Look, you have His saving grace anyway because you are a human being, a good person and full of love, not only for yourself but first of all for those close to you, even your enemies, isn't that so?

Costas nodded a yes.

— Now, for as long as you are with us, as I said earlier, you will allow us to keep you alive on this earth, in our way, and with all our might, so that your body can function in the best possible way...

... In every way we know. Those ways too have been granted us By Divine Grace and Providence. It is something we don't dispute. You will take the medication we give you, and have a chat with your doctor, Mr. Papadopoulos, every day. Twice a week all of us together will review your state of health.

— But I already told you there's nothing wrong with me. I'm fine. And, as I said, I'm not going to take any of your medicine.

— And in turn I told you that is the one thing that isn't up for negotiation. If you won't take it, we'll have to inject you. I don't think you want to act like a little child, you can see our side of it. You are our responsibility.

The psychiatrist's first duty is to speak the language of the patient sitting there in front of him. This means he or she must share in the schizophrenic's delusions, using arguments that agree with theirs. In the case of Costas, the religious arguments helped to convince him more easily. In other instances, where patients think they are hunted by secret services who are interfering with their brain and thought processes in some way, I tell them the medication I shall give them will strengthen their brain, to make them less vulnerable. Maybe I also give them the excuse they need so as to accept what may not be avoided, which is to take their medication.

The second element necessary for communication with a schizophrenic is that the psychiatrist must make it clear <u>from the start</u> that certain things such as taking the medication are not to be bargained with. The clearer and unequivocal the situation, the less there will be clashes. If a margin for argument is allowed either by the doctor or the nursing staff, it is to be expected that a patient encountering these conditions for the first time will try to counter our decisions. Our attitude too, must be as clearly definite and imperturbable so as not to allow space for equivocation.

I always remember my first experience with a severely paranoid schizophrenic when I was new to my residency in psychiatry. Like every young dissenter, when my professor told me to administer a patient's treatment forcibly by injection, I jumped up and said that I would try to persuade him to take the medication by mouth, to avoid injecting him by force. My professor, an experienced psychiatrist, took a good look at me and said: "Have a go and we'll see …"

Sure enough, two hours later of trying to convince the patient who wouldn't take his medication, I had reached my limit and my arguments' limit too. My patience was also at an end and so was his. So, the arrogance of youth knocked out of me, I had to go shamefacedly to beg for assistance from the nurses. There was a struggle over the injection because in the meanwhile the patient had become enraged. As long as he thought there was a margin allowing him to reject the medicine and space for transaction, he became more pressing. It consequently became more difficult to persuade him. It has ever since been a lesson for me. The signposting has to be clear and the message transmitted from the start: "certain things are not to be negotiated."

In this case, Costas accepted my treatment because he realised that if he refused, it would be given by injection. And he got better by the day. Communication with his saint became less intensive. For hours at a time he heard less audible delusions, and with time, even for days. He became less delusionary and their impact lost their intensity. He no longer spoke of nothing but his communication with the Divine and was more cooperative. He was coming back more to the real world and gradually emerging from the world of delusion. He talked to his fellow patients and the staff and gave up fasting, burning incense and praying. At first, alone in his room, he had incense burning all the time as he murmured prayers, but a week later he was conscious of the danger of his habit as a fire risk for the clinic and stopped it, together with the constant praying.

A month later, he no longer heard the voice of the saint.

– *How do you explain this, Costas?*

– *Evidently, God understood that in here it isn't necessary. Nor should He guided me. I think that when I go home I will get the contact back.*

– *You exclude the possibility that the medication might have stopped the voices?*

– *Come on, how could the medicine you give have chased away Saint Anthony? No, no way.*

– *But suppose the saint's voice was coming from inside you? Supposing it was the effect of your great faith, that short–circuited in your brain so that your thoughts transformed into an external voice? Because if that's what happened it explains that it stopped because of the medication. The medication untangled your brain and broke the short circuit. That's how you stopped hearing the voice, which you think is Saint Anthony's but which is apparently expressing your own innate fears, hopes and aspirations.*

– *But, Doctor, I could hear it so clearly!*

– *Just as you hear mine now. That's how it is. It wasn't your imagination. Or rather, it was your imagination, which because of the short–circuit in your brain made it sound as if it was coming to your ears. There's no magic about it. It's something very simple. A mechanical fault, I could call it, that's corrected by the medicine you're taking.*

– *You mean, if I stop them I'll hear it again?*

– *Not straight away. Not from the first day you won't take your medication. But a few weeks, a few months later it will come back for sure. If you do stop taking the medicine, in fact, at the beginning you may even feel better, because you won't feel the side effects the treatment usually has. Don't stop taking them. You need them.*

– *Doctor! What are you telling me? That I have to take them forever? That's impossible!*

– *And why so? How come I've been taking medicine for my thyroid that isn't functioning properly, for the last ten years? And as a matter of fact, I know I'll be taking it until I die. There's nothing strange about it. Nearly everybody nowadays is taking some sort of medication; some for blood pressure, some for blood sugar, there are even those who have a daily injection of insulin. What should they say? What's more, we ought to be grateful that there is treatment so we can live healthier lives. Without them most of us would be dead. In fact, science today is going a step further, focusing on preventive medicine. I've been taking medicine for the last ten years that lowers cholesterol because I believe it will delay coronary artery plaque so that maybe I won't have a heart attack! Is that crazy? Yet not only I am doing it, there are millions of us, intelligent people, in a civilized world.*

I give this little speech to all my patients to persuade them to keep taking their medication. It is usually successful because it puts what they have to take for their mental ailment on a par with the more usual treatments. It lessens the stigma that for all of us exists as to mental illness and any 'drug' – a term I avoid at all costs — that affects the mind. That's because the term is used in a most derogatory and besmirching sense, for a whole category of pharmaceuticals that in fact save lives. Let us just think that until 1950 when anti-psychotic medication was discovered, schizophrenics were simply imprisoned, in asylums which were called psychiatric clinics. Nowadays though, most of them do not only live freely in the community, they have jobs; they marry and lead a relatively normal life. If we bear this in mind, we should have deep respect for these medicines and not disparage them.

– *Does that mean, Doctor, that I am never going to get better?*

– *You will get better, but to stay well you will have to take them always. Most people have to have continued treatment. Yet, I don't complain about my thyroid problem. I say it's o.k. because I take a pill every morning and the blood tests that I have regularly, are normal.*

This is where the game is played with each patient: how to persuade them to take their medication as consistently as possible. A good doctor is one who does not only make his patients better, but also maintains them in good health. I tell my students that every day I see patients who have seen other colleagues and have been furnished with excellent prescriptions. But they come to me, because obviously they did not follow the prescription correctly or maybe have not even started taking the recommended medication. Why not? Because the doctor didn't convince them. They didn't trust him. He didn't look them straight in the eye. They thought he didn't listen to them or didn't take them seriously.

Medicine is a difficult Art. Knowledge is not enough. It also needs skill to win over the patient, to win their trust. To convince him to do as you say. That is how to be a successful doctor. Otherwise, if you think about it, nowadays the entire body of knowledge can be found in the Internet. However, the more the information is diffused, the more it loses its credibility. There is no way accessibility to information can be a substitute for a doctor, rather the contrary, more information leads more people to see a doctor. Of a good doctor, who will manage to gain their confidence, guide them to a correct diagnosis and, above all, to the most suitable therapy for them. Good doctors have nothing to fear from informatics. Fortunately or unfortunately, there will always 'be a shortage' of good doctors!

Schizophrenia: a biological illness

WHOEVER HAS taught medical students has met with doubting of the definition of mental disease and pathological behaviour. It is often difficult to convince young people – who are usually objectors– that a person should be classed as ill because they hear voices that nobody else hears and who believe they communicate with God or that they are followed by secret servicemen.

Nevertheless, schizophrenia is not a personal choice, nor is it a social phenomenon but an illness, in fact found the world over. It is an illness with about the same frequency in all societies, from the most capitalist and Westernised to the most primitive in the depth of the jungle, steadily fluctuating at about 1.5% of the population.

There is also something else: schizophrenia has a hereditary side to it. It means that we know today that a person from a family with a history of schizophrenia is more likely to suffer from it than someone who does not have a schizophrenic relative. If therefore the general public has a 1.5% possibility of having the disorder, when somebody has a parent or sibling with schizophrenia the odds rise to 14%. This is irrespective of the family in whom we grew up, since it has been found in siblings who were adopted into different families. They had the same chances of having the illness whether they had grown up in their own, biological family or in a family with no history of schizophrenia.

On the other hand, studies with identical twins, that is from the same egg with identical genetic material proved that the cause of schizophrenia is not only hereditary, as only 50% of the identical siblings of schizophrenics developed the illness. That is, half the siblings did not suffer from the illness whilst the other, genetically identical, had it. This shows that something else beside the gene provokes the sickness to declare itself.

It is however another element that has no relation to the environment and the pressure this may exert on the person prone to the disease. Twins are treated the same way by their family as well as by the school and the broader community, since in fact they often cannot be told apart especially when they are both dressed the same. This means that when schizophrenia declares itself it has nothing to do with the upbringing or social pressure the person may have.

I stress this because it is important for parents of schizophrenics not to feel guilty, nor think it may be their fault if their child has the illness. In particular we should be aware that guilt feelings are the worst state of mind in which to confront this chronic illness.

Parents must not feel guilty because it is not their fault in any way; to blame is the transmission of genes. But then short people, or the bald or short-sighted or diabetics should feel guilty too. It is the rule in the propagation of species. We all of us carry 'pathological' as well as 'ameliorating' genes, that will transmit their properties to our descendants only when they are crossed with corresponding genes of the other parent.

To come back to schizophrenia: the appearance or not of the illness in identical twins must be due to the difference of neuronal routes that the brain of one of the twins has selected to activate whereas the brain of the other, apparently randomly, preferred another route for the processing of these exact stimulations. In this way one brain opened a faulty channel, with the result that when at the age of 17 or 20 a large quantity of stimulations passed through this 'channel', the short–circuits will occur, about which I shall have more to say below.

An interesting model

IN THE last few years I have been using a simplifying model for the benefit of my students that describes the principle mental pathology demonstrated in schizophrenia using computer terminology. The familiarity of young people with computers helps the model to be assimilated, making it more attractive.

To be precise, I say that there is a 'Central Processor' in our brain that processes the data it receives from diverse sources, based on which it produces decisions and conclusions. This 'Central Processor' receives data on the one hand from the 'External Environment', that is different sensory sources: optical, audible, olfactory and others, channeled to it through specific entrances (these are called gates or ports in computers). On the other hand, the 'Central Processor' receives data from another processor as well, which I call 'Thought'. 'Thought' produces data from elements stored in the past, from convictions that have been formed, in general, data sent to it earlier from the 'Central Processor'.

'Thought's' data are channeled to the 'Central Processor' by a specific and different entrance from the one used by those coming from the 'External Environment'. Thus the 'Central Processor' knows that if some data come to it from 'Thought's entrance, it means it is a product of its own thought, its own imagination. If on the contrary it comes from the entrance of data from the 'External Environment', it recognises them as real, that is, data from the external reality.

It is therefore easy to understand that if there is a short–circuit and data from 'Thought' is channeled to the 'Central Processor' through the 'External' entrance,

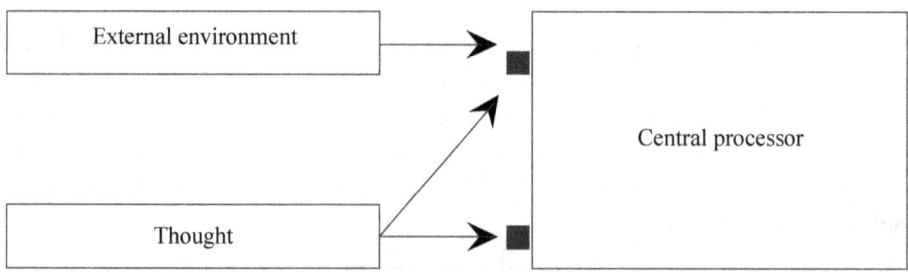

the 'Central Processor' will think they are coming from the outside world. This is how auditory delusions are formed, whose content expresses our own thoughts, our fears, and whatever else comes out of the processor of 'Thought'.

For instance, if someone who is very religious fervently wishes to communicate with God and the saints and this wish enters into his brain's 'Central Processor' from the gate/port the external stimuli come through, the 'Central Processor' will think he is truly hearing the voice of God or of the saints. If it entered through the right gate/port they will recognise that they are their own thoughts and wishes and therefore not real.

This model helps to see that the obvious therapy for this brain disorder is to disrupt the short–circuits, which are affected by administration of anti–psychotic drugs.

My theory of short–circuits is to explain the pathogenic cause of schizophrenia even to the patients themselves and their family. A number of patients are persuaded by it to take the treatment as well as accept the chronicity of the treatment. It also frees the parents from feelings of guilt since I explain that it is not their fault nor is it because of the way they brought up the patient. I tell them that there is probably some inherited vulnerability to this defect, for which they are, of course, not to blame.

It is my firm conviction that the more the scientific facts concerning the sickness are made known to society so that mental illness is no different from a biological disease, the more the stigma attached to schizophrenia and the other states will diminish. It is not necessary to campaign against the stigma, it disappears itself when society is informed of the advances of modern psychiatry. This is what happened with tuberculosis, popularly stigmatised in many places. As soon as an effective antibiotic treatment was discovered in 1949, the stain cast on the tubercular patients, even on their families, disappeared as by magic.

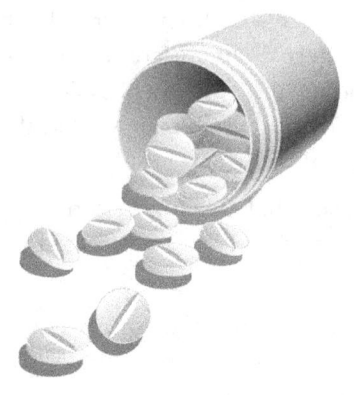

THE PATIENT'S COMPLIANCE AND HIS/HER PERSONAL RESPONSIBILITY

– *Doctor, I feel so much better now that they aren't after me and I don't hear the people around me making comments about me.*

– *I'm very glad to hear it. You see that in the end you did have to take the medication the doctors prescribed for you... They were right.*

– *I don't know if they were right. What I do know is that now I don't hear voices in my head any more, my brain is clear.*

– *But to stay clear, young man, I have to insist that you keep taking your medicine absolutely regularly.*

– *So you say. But I think I know now what was wrong with me. I've understood what I didn't realise and my brain is never going to get mixed up again.*

– *Let me make this quite clear: it is not up to you. It is only thanks to the medication that you got better and are in a good state now. If you stop taking it, I'm warning you, you will relapse. And that means starting from scratch, all over again. Hospitalisation against your will, treatment with medicines ... and if you're lucky your brain may get to the point where it is today.*

– *O.k., o.k., Doctor... all of you are geared to medicines.*

– I can't put it any other way. This is it: stopping the treatment results in relapse!

Unfortunately, despite the best efforts, in most cases the outcome is predictable. Schizophrenics nearly always stop their therapy and 80% of them at least relapse within a few months!

I attended a discussion at a psychiatric conference recently on the subject of the compliance of the mentally ill with their treatment. What surprised me is that we professionals in the field of mental health have accepted the 'irresponsibility' of our patients. It is the psychiatrist, together with the parents, who feel responsible for continuation of the cooperation between patient and doctor.

In my long experience as a psychiatrist I have often come to be exasperated, and in fact infuriated, by schizophrenics who while taking their medication and were in a good state of health, arbitrarily diminished the dosage or ceased the therapy, with the inevitable result that they relapsed. I cannot therefore accept that when a patient is completely reasonable, meaning they are fully conscious of having an illness and that he is free of psychopathology and symptoms, he may be considered irresponsible.

I believe on the contrary that they are just as responsible as the diabetic, for whom the doctor has prescribed a diet and meticulous testing for blood sugar, and who neglects it. The diabetic is just as responsible for the resulting angiopathy (disease of the blood vessels), generally followed by amputation, in just the same way that the schizophrenic inevitably ends up being forcibly sectioned.

The illness does not even give the schizophrenic an alibi, because generally, when they stop their therapy and break the medical contract, they are capable of perceiving that this cessation will result in a relapse. They may be aware of it, but unfortunately do not believe it will happen to them. In the same way smokers realise the consequence of the habit but basically believe that they will 'get away with it'.

It makes me so angry that in Greece thousands of amputations are performed each year on diabetics, or when I think of the prevalence of chronic pulmonary obstructive disease, of lung cancer and heart attacks due to smoking. Well, to tell you the truth, I am just as angered by the 'revolving doors' of psychiatric clinics. I mean, to see patients leaving in good health and shortly after returning, sick again. It is not my colleagues I am angry at, but human nature that makes us preposterous and superficial. Because, it may be said, it is foolish and frivolous to disregard the prescriptions of Science, which derive from quantities of experimental observations and research data.

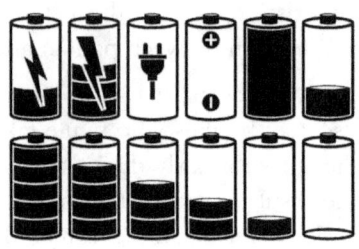

DEPRESSION: THE BATTERY NEEDS RECHARGING

ALL THE epidemiological studies show that this disorder that we call 'depression' is appearing ever more frequently. In the 'civilised' world the numbers are climbing year by year, with no sign of diminution. Pharmaceutical companies were rubbing their hands. Their clientele is assured and, in fact, increasing. However, unfortunately for the major multi-nationals pharmaceutical companies, excellent antidepressant drugs were produced during the 90's, which have now lost their patents so that their price drops day by day.

More than 5% of the population of the USA today takes antidepressants. In locations such as New York the frequency is greater. Most people will soon have to take antidepressants after a certain age and for a long stretch of time.

Is that harsh? Maybe, but quite realistic. Just as a large portion of the population living in areas where there is a surplus of food take statins, drugs that reduce cholesterol, in the same way those living where life races ahead with speed, will have to take antidepressants.

Today we know that depression is due to exhaustion of a neuron circuit in the brain, possibly a serotonergic circuit, that is to say mainly having a malfunctioning serotonin connection. The neurons constituting it are exhausted and no longer function satisfactorily.

This knowledge, as most often happens in medicine, did not result from organised and planned research but from observations of chance events. Some perceptive clinical physicians observed that tubercular patients who were taking a specific medicine were happier, and in fact those who were depressive improved as by magic. The then saw that one of the properties of this medicine, isoniazid, was to increase the serotonin and noradrenaline in the brain. Pharmacologists therefore tried to fabricate special drugs that would mainly provoke the increase of these substances in the brain and tried them on patients suffering from depression. The results were unprecedented for the times.

We need only think that until 1960 there was no special therapy for depression. Patients were dealt with by encouragement and psychological support. Some psychiatrists and psychologists attempted to find what brought patients to such a state. They sought traumas in their childhood in the hope that if the patients were helped to overcome them they might be reprieved from the depression that troubled them.

However, when antidepressants were discovered, all the data known to date were overturned. A psychiatrist could now, within a few days or weeks, make a depressive person who saw everything around them in shades of black and no way out anywhere, enjoy life and be smiling again. What's more, this dramatic change takes place with no psychotherapeutic intervention, no change in the surroundings of the patient. With no alteration in the least of the circumstances that brought about the depression. It is simply that antidepressants make someone see things more optimistically. They 'reset' the tendency to see everything pessimistically, dark and at a dead end.

– I cannot fathom how I had sunk to such a low point, Doctor! How I had drowned. I could think of nothing but the loss of my father. Not even the children's presence made me happy. I wanted to be alone in bed or on the sofa, to think … of unpleasant things only. And dead ends, dead ends everywhere.

Obviously, antidepressants do not alter reality. What they succeed in doing is to retrieve the normal breadth of the filters of the thought process which, because of depression, had shrunk down to pessimistic thoughts only. That is to say that depression restricts the brain's filters of search to fields of exploration of depressing issues alone. After treatment, typically, many depressives say they when they were in depression they could think nothing but black and pessimistic thoughts and scenarios.

When antidepressants were discovered, it was indisputable that depression was too a biological disease. A disorder of a circuit in the brain. The exhaustion of a particular serotonergic circuit. What antidepressants do is enable the serotonergic neurons to function without loss. In this way their normal operation is restored as the drugs make the function of these neurons more inexpensive i.e. without 'leakage' and thus more efficient. This is why antidepressants are not immediately effective: it is simply because they are helping the troubled neurons to recover.

There are, of course, patients whose circuit is exhausted to the point of being unable to recover without continuing medication support. It is evident that they will need antidepressant treatment for life.

What I have learnt from experience is that the same thing happens in depression as in schizophrenia, which is to say that after every relapse the next phase is more difficult to treat. It needs increased dosage of medication and longer time to work.

A patient of mine noticed this first:

– How is it possible that I am taking so much medicine and am still no better? The last time I was depressed, after a disappointment in love, when I was 19, crying inconsolably and unable to sleep, our family doctor gave me some tranquilizers and after a week I was fine. When I came to you five years ago, aged forty, when I was depressed again after my father's sudden death, you gave me 20mg of antidepressants and I was fit as a fiddle in a couple of weeks. Now that my husband has had to close his shop and we are in a difficult financial state, you prescribed triple the dose and I still don't see any improvement…

This particular patient did get better after a fortnight, but in order to get her into good condition I had to add another, stronger, antidepressant. In fact, for just the reason she had told me, I recommended she did not stop her drug therapy. However, a few months later, when she was reconciled to her new circumstances, she gradually stopped the treatment.

She was back a year later, in tears. Her child had had an accident – minor, fortunately – but being particularly sensitive, she became depressed again. Before even calling me, from previous experience, she had of herself begun treatment. But this time, it necessitated a combination of two different antidepressants, at maximum dosage, reinforced with some lithium, a favourite cocktail of mine, to get the patient out of her depression. After this she did not dare stop, nor even diminish her treatment on her own initiative.

It therefore appears that when the circuit responsible for depression is exhausted once, it is more easily exhausted again, even in situations of lesser stress. Furthermore, every exhaustion of the circuit makes its recharging more difficult. It is in a way like a battery which, the more often they are recharged, the more difficult it is to charge them. This why after a certain point constant pharmaceutical underpinning of the circuit becomes inevitable.

Three factors cause depression:

• First that the inherited circuitry is of medium or poor quality.

• Second, that the circumstances of mental stress we are under are excessive, that is that our brain is under strain from too many events exerting pressure on it. Too many decisions to make. Too many reversals in life which, in fact it should be known, have an exponential effect. Patients often tell me that the last event before depression set in was not all that significant, as was what had happened in the past. But it seems that the latest event was the cherry on the cake, before it collapsed.

• Third, in direct relation to the second, when our character, our personality, provokes an excessive over–function of that circuit. That is to wish for perfection in everything to the degree of becoming anxious about things that others do not normally find anguishing. When one is a perfectionist to the point of details being insufferable.

Also this is the point at which psychotherapy can intervene since genes cannot be altered, nor can the external circumstances of life that are stressful. Consequently, all that can be done is to become a little more insensitive, not to be anguished about any minor thing that happens to us, especially when there is nothing to be done about it. Even worse, of course, is that many people are afraid that something could happen to them.

One should therefore try to change one's character, even a little bit. Obviously, it isn't easy to change the way we deal with situations significantly. All that can be hoped for is that even a small change might protect us from some mental stress which could play a crucial role in burdening that particular neural circuit.

In any case, to encourage my patients to make a change, I underline the fact that it is their perfectionism that is at fault and brought on the depression. If they do not change the way they deal with their problems, they will need to be reinforced with medication all their life.

— *Some people lose sleep over a fender–bender, while others get over a serious collision calmly, saying 'never mind, it's only metal, it will be repaired… as long as we are o.k.' A little superficiality is necessary to get through life's reverses. Be a bit more thick–skinned, do not let every little thing get to you and particularly, hurt you.*

— *But, Doctor, I can't change! I can see it for myself but it's beyond my powers.*

— *In that case the alternative is to leave the demanding life you lead and go and live where there will be fewer demands made on your mental state. Quit your job in the brokers' firm, since you can't handle it, and go and become a fisherman on some island. That way, instead of your brain having to process thousands of imponderables and factors difficult to control, all you'll have to think about will be the weather. Is it fair? You'll go out fishing. Is it too rough? You stay at home. Simplicity!*

Depression: a gift from modern life

IT IS EVIDENT that the human brain was not constructed to bear the excessive uses it is subjected to by those who live at the rhythm of our consumer society. One needs only to think that, until two generations ago, the data to be processed by the brain was minimal compared to what it has to do nowadays.

Nobody asked my grandmother what she thought of my grandfather, who was to be her husband. She was not asked her opinion, nor was that of any of her girlfriends. The girls just knew that they would marry the man their parents would 'find' for them. Even today, in many parts of the world, women get married without the groom having ever so much as seen them. Needless to say that in some places they wear a burkha and no male has ever seen their face. So they don't need to look beautiful or be slender, blonde, to work out, remove body hair, to wear make–up and scent. There is, you see, a good side to the burkha!

Any woman can easily see the quantities of data that her brain processes every day, so as to be as pretty and as attractive as possible for the opposite sex: what to wear that is fashionable and suit her figure? What make–up and which perfume? Let alone the dilemma of making a choice: whom to select and how to get close to him, what tactics to use to get him to notice her and finally to attract him? Should she be talkative in company, or not? And say what? Something clever, or would that be rushing things and be misinterpreted? Should she propose going to the cinema, or what about a drink in a bar? Is she pushing or, if she doesn't act will it be seen as indifference? Play hard to get or might that lose her the interest of the prospective candidate for her love or future bridegroom?

None of all these bothered my grandmother. Neither was my grandfather bothered, by all that preoccupies the male of today. Here is an ordinary example: driving to Kifissia in the northern suburbs of Athens, in a hurry as usual, I wonder:

— Shall I change lanes, because this one seems to be slow? The next driver on my left doesn't seem disposed to let me in front of him. Shall I force things, using my indicator lights and swerving abruptly left? He might swear at me, and he would be right, but I'm in such a hurry! Shall I stay in my queue? Or shall I let him past and change lanes the next time there is a gap?

Within the space of two minutes, my brain has had to solve dilemmas my ancestors did not encounter in years. Most of them had only one concern: to return from grazing with the same number of sheep. They had left the pen with ten in the morning. Ten had to be brought back in the afternoon. That was all. Or they cast their nets and caught some quantity of fish. It was what God had sent them and they had no other choice.

The options of today's 'modern' man are exorbitant and there are more of them every day. It is these options that exhaust the power of the processor function. They exhaust the serotonergic neural circuit, which is what provokes depression when it malfunctions.

Fortunately, concurrently with the complication of life, man discovered antidepressants that reinforce the functioning of the processor so that they can manage. Antidepressants are like spectacles for presbyopia. If they did not exist, most of us would be 'finished' from the age of forty. We would not be able to read or write, we would be sitting on a couch telling our grandchildren stories or doing some rough chores for as long as our bodily strength allowed. If we want to stay active in our modern times, we have to wear spectacles.

In 'Uzala', Kurosawa's wonderful film, when the primitive man of the same name in the leading role grows old and can no longer aim his weapon to hunt, he decides to die since he is useless according to the laws of nature. This is how all of nature operates. Modern man alone can remedy the ravages of time and his physiological defects. Just as the short–sighted can participate in all modern activities, in the same way, those who need antidepressants can go on leading their life with the same intensity, thanks to them.

Continuing use of antidepressants is not an addiction to something useless, like smoking. It is an imperative search for help. The alternative solution for those sufferers is to give up the life they lead and live a less demanding lifestyle, to simplify it; to go and become fishermen, or farmers, or herdsmen in the traditional way. I say 'traditional', because nowadays even fishermen go fishing with an ultrasonic fishing device and consult weather reports. They even analyse data for prices of their produce. Farming too has become a science needing constant updating.

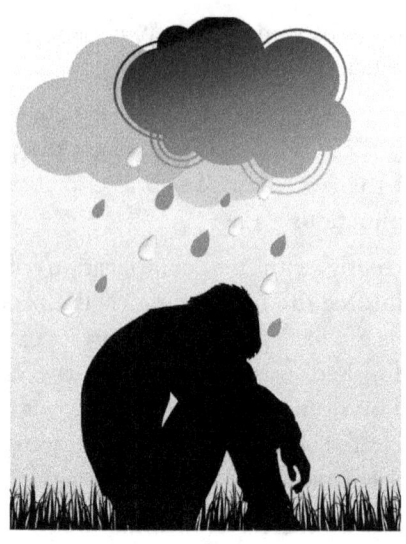

RECESSION AND DEPRESSION

THE OTHER DAY a man of about forty, whose name is Lefteris, came in to see me to ask for a prescription for the persistent sleeplessness he had suffered from all the previous month. Barely had I begun questioning him about the causes of his insomnia when with tears in his eyes and a breaking voice as he spoke, he started telling me his personal troubles, behaving as if he were defending himself before an invisible tribunal:

— I did nothing wrong… I was neither unreasonable nor careless… I'm not a crook. But all of a sudden I feel like the worst of criminals, who has to pay for the crimes he committed …

His story came rushing out in a flood. All I could do was to show by my attitude that I was listening to him with keen interest. I took care not to interrupt, even when he paused. When he turned to me I looked him in the eyes, sometimes leaning in towards him, so as to encourage him.

— … I was one of the most successful salesmen in a big car showroom. I worked there for ten years and no one ever had anything to complain of. The last years I was earning 4,000 Euros a month. I went to work every morning, I never shirked… My wife too was making money. She was manager in a boutique, and she too was on her feet all day… Two years ago, as our daughter was about to start school, we decided to move away from my family home in Nea Liossia (a working-class neighborhood). We took out a loan to buy a flat in Maroussi a

chic suburb, where there are good schools and it's also closer to both our workplaces… We did nothing foolish. The interest on the mortgage was 2,000 Euros a month, while I was making 4,000 and my wife 3,000. And we were getting 400 a month in rent from my old house … We enrolled our little girl in a good school and gave thanks to the Lord… but we didn't get a chance to enjoy our happiness. The bottom fell out of our life in the last six months. You probably know that car sales have fallen, well, to cut a long story short, the showroom closed down and, you see, there's no way I can find work in that sector any more. I went round to all the car sales agencies to enquire, but nobody is hiring. They're laying people off everywhere. There's no point in trudging around all day with my CV in my hand. You can't imagine how desperate every day makes me. I wear a suit and tie and go around the whole area, putting a fat smile on my face but there's a black dog on my back. Every day that goes by, the smile is more forced and false. However good a salesman I may be, I can't sell myself any more. It's useless and saddening… The sadness is growing and it's choking me.

Lefteris broke down and sobbed. I bent over and gave him a tissue. My expression showed all the compassion I was feeling, in the true sense of the word 'sympathy'. Because I was really suffering for this poor man's plight, a man with so much ambition, so decent and hard working. Believe me, it's hard to see a proud fellow crying like that!

— *… All the time I was going around looking for work was a torment. I've stopped now. There isn't any point.*

— *What about your wife?*

— *Oh Doctor, I can't tell you how bad it is. It's as if we were being hounded by the Furies. Two months ago the boutique where she was working also closed… But she has connections and good relations with her customers she looked after so well and she managed to find a job as an ordinary salesgirl in a boutique in the big shopping mall. Her salary is 1,500 Euros and we're grateful for it… The bank rings me every day. I can't pay the interest on the mortgage … We're going to lose our home … There's no way out. We'll have to go back to my family house… Every time I look around our flat it's as though I'm seeing it for the last time. I feel like someone condemned to death.*

— *Oh come now,* — I said. — *It's not as bad as that! Lots of people have had to move. It isn't the end of the world. And, you know, nothing lasts forever.*

— *And what are we supposed to say to our child? It's not myself and my wife I feel so bad about. She understands… But to tell you the truth, Doctor, as man to man you can understand me too: however often she says that she understands, I'm sure that in her inner self she must be despising me. She goes off to work every morning. The child goes to school and I … I do the housework. Doctor, I can't go on. I feel it's my responsibility. I'm the head of the household, it's the man's job to provide for his family… That's how we were brought up. And of course, it's me the bank is after. I feel so useless. And at the same time so helpless. There's nothing I can do to avoid disaster. This is what goes round and round in my head at night, and I simply can't sleep...*

It was time for me to intervene, and what's more, energetically. We had reached the final stage. According to my preferred tactics, instead of using words of comfort and sympathy, I became confrontational, and may perhaps have sounded a bit aggressive:

— That's enough self-flagellation. After all, you said it yourself, you've done nothing wrong. And so what, there's a crisis and a recession, because of which you lost your job — it isn't your fault. There's a war going on out there but you didn't start it. You have to get that into your head. You are simply a victim of the circumstances. And just as in war, if your house is bombed you'll say 'thank the Lord': that my family and I survived. Even if you lose home and hearth, furniture and all... you'll take your child in your arms and with your wife, you'll go to the old family home, which is still standing and be grateful that you have a shelter for them, a roof over your family's head. That's how it is today. We all of us have to come to terms with it.

— Yes, but, Doctor, not everyone is in my situation!

— Not yet... But don't think we are not all hit by the crisis. Not all the houses have been destroyed but everybody feels the pinch. Anyway, even in a bombardment not all the houses are demolished. You're lucky, you have somewhere to go. Some people are living in their car. You know they are... And when they bought their car from you, they didn't think for a moment that anything like that might happen to them.

I had to lighten up a little, be less severe. While at the same time telling him that others were in a worse state.

— The fact that there's worse, — he said — doesn't make things any easier for me.

— True, but it doesn't mean you have the right to moan that the sky fell on your head. It happened to all of us, some more and some less. In any case, what you have to be conscious of is that your personal responsibilities are minimal. You have no cause for remorse and feelings of guilt.

— Oh, am I supposed to be happy about things then?

— No, I'm not saying that, but if you realise that it's a general problem and that it isn't because of you, you'll look forward, ahead, and stop whining about what you lost. Do you know, during the war and the occupation, people did not let themselves sink into depression. They lost all their money, loved ones were killed, but the survivors looked ahead. They saw to their subsistence until the war was over. The war <u>will</u> end, some time. It's the only sure thing. If we get through it, we'll enjoy the fruits of peace. Even the history of economics tells of cycles of boom and bust. What happened is that after a time of easy growth and the bubble that went with it, it burst and came down on our head. It was obvious. It's just that nobody knew when it would happen. That's the way things are.

I took a deep breath. He was looking at me, he seemed a little relieved. Also, perhaps, perplexed; what I was saying was all too obvious, yet he hadn't thought about it that way. Not, at least, in that dimension. I continued my 'sermon':

— *We are the first generation in this country that has not experienced a war. In fact, you, who are younger, did not even hear the vivid stories we were told as we grew up. When I was a boy, every day my parents were telling me about the occupation. I grew up with the 'occupation syndrome'. I was ashamed not to 'eat up all my food' or to throw out something that 'could come in useful someday'! Of course in those days the notion of recycling didn't exist, but my mother couldn't throw away so much as a bottle, 'in case we need it one day', as she would always say to me. If ever I protested, she would repeat, again and again, "you haven't been through the occupation — and I hope you never have to ..."*

— *And are you saying that it is here now, Doctor?*

— *It isn't here in the sense my mother meant. But this recession is showing us that life can't always be easy. There will be ups and downs, things will go topsy–turvy. In 1929 my grandfather was a tobacco merchant and owned warehouses, and then, overnight, he had to become a humble grocer. He will have sighed for his lost fortune but he managed to survive and he provided for his family — seven children! I think we have forgotten everything the past taught us. You'd think all we learned from history was not about humankind but some extra–terrestrials. We wanted to think we were living in a fairyland, a magic place where nothing could touch us. But, I'm afraid that's not reality. We thought our generation, and yours to follow us, would escape 'the treadmill of History'. But it was too good to be true. Don't worry, we'll get over this. In any case, it looks as if history merely grazed us.*

— *You're an optimist, Doctor. You may be right, but I don't care about myself... It's what do I tell my daughter? How can I face her? How can I look into her eyes and tell her she has to change schools? She doesn't know anything about history and economic cycles.*

— *But it's precisely for her and her generation that it will be the best lesson. Lessons are learned best in practice, not in theory. That was exactly the trouble with your generation. You were taught the theory, so you never believed you could ever confront anything like it, whereas I heard it at firsthand and somehow it concerned me more intimately. I heard the whine of bullets in my ears. You, however, and your contemporaries have been sitting on the comfortable couch that modern Greek society has made for you. Wars were far away and you saw them as a product of TV that had nothing to do with your daily existence. Even when you were watching the bombing of Yugoslavia, a little further up in our neighborhood, for most of you it was a myth, a montage for the newsreels. Like something contrary to the laws of nature, something unreasonable, metaphysical. We all thought the words 'war', 'devastation', even the word 'poverty' were not part of the life we were leading. Our generations had acquired a permanent immunity to them. As if the Marshall Plan for Europe was a miraculous vaccine. We were all vaccinated with 'progress' and 'prosperity'.*

— *It's true, I never heard anything about this from my parents. Everywhere all the time*

I heard only that all would be well. Even any failure of mine seemed temporary and would be forgotten. There were always alternative solutions. Now that I think of it, even my failing the university entrance exams turned out well for me, because an uncle found me this job in car sales and I started earning money from the age of eighteen. Well, of course, I can't say ... I washed cars and swept the salesroom for the early years, but I always had more pocket money that my friends who were students. And, not to be ungrateful, for the past ten years I have been earning a good salary, as has my wife. It's just that as you said, Doctor, we didn't expect things to go wrong.

– Don't worry, it isn't the end of the world. Not only are we going to survive, but in 20 years' time you will be telling your children and your grandchildren about all this like a story of heroism. Just as our parents and grandparents were heroes. You know, difficulties are easily forgotten, and the passage of time makes them even appear ... as nostalgia!

At the end of our talk, Lefteris seemed relieved of the load that was crushing him. With the help of some antidepressant drug I recommended, he came out of the defeatism and hopelessness which had brought him to me. He told me two months later that he had reached a better settlement with his bank and managed to keep his flat. He also found a job driving a truck and he and his wife are doing their best.

Unfortunately, Lefteris's story is not unique but it does show that it's all a matter of the subjective approach to things. No situation is ever a dead–end. Even the worst calamity has a way out and a new life thereafter. History never stands still.

Very often, in fact, the way out may be close by, but we cannot see it, simply because we do not turn our head to look. We are frequently stuck in a particular direction and wait there to see the 'light at the end of the tunnel', from that spot alone.

A lady between forty and fifty years old came to my office in despair. Her husband was a pensioned civil servant whose pension was getting less every day. She had two sons, 22 and 25 years old, unemployed. She was in a state of panic, what she saw ahead of her was a Calvary with her three men... crucified.

– Every day at home is like a funeral. Nobody says anything. We just look at one another and try to hide our desperation.

– And you all live off your husband's pension?

– Yes, exactly, Doctor. As you can imagine, we just about manage to make ends meet. After buying cigarettes and giving the boys their pocket money, there's nothing left. If as they say, my husband's pension is reduced even more, what's going to happen to us then?

– O.k., but what do your sons say about it?

– What should they say? The older one had a job as a graphics artist in an advertising

agency, but as you know agencies are closing down one after another, so not only did he lose his job but he can't find another. He sits at home and waits for the crisis to pass. And that's not all, you see, Doctor ... he can't find a girlfriend either. He's had the wind taken out of his sails. This also reflects on the younger one ... As I said, it's all gloom and doom at home.

— *What was the younger one's job?*

— *He had some training in electronics and worked in a shop selling computers. Unfortunately that closed too and the young one was out of work too. Both my children are unemployed and no future prospects anywhere...*

When things look black, my mind reacts vigorously. It will not accept defeat and seeks to hang on to details like some demon detective. The lady's surname was from a northern part of Greece but her accent was typical Cretan, which is what I latched onto.

— *Where are you from? I asked her.*

— *From Crete... what about it?*

— *Do you have any links there? Do you visit often?*

— *Yes, of course I do, Doctor. In fact since my husband was pensioned, he's been pestering me to move to Chania (Crete's second largest town) where I have a house. Although he isn't from Crete he's tired of Athens and has a better time with my relatives in Chania.*

— *Well, why don't the boys look for work in Crete. The tourist trade is doing well there and they aren't in recession. And if your sons can't find work in their field they'll be able to do something else. Where there's a will there's a way...*

I said this just to show her that everything was not at such an impasse as she made it out to be, but to be honest I didn't think my advice would have such good results. As it was, four months later she was back to ask for another prescription and for me to 'tell her how to quit the antidepressants drugs'. She told me with pride that her elder son was already working in a graphics arts company in Chania and the younger was going to be employed in the same company, creating Internet sites for tourist enterprises in the area. The mother I saw before me was a different person from the anguished and desperate woman I had seen a few months earlier.

Telling of this case brings me to a phenomenon, or rather a misrepresentation I have come across several times. Parents are carried away by the movement trumpeting the freedom of choice for children, which has had the most adverse effect on the post–war generations, and let their children make decisions 'freely' as to their studies and professional orientation. The result of this 'freedom of choice' is to have filled our country with a host of unemployed degree holders, young people who have wasted their best years studying useless sciences.

Typical instances I have seen in recent years are legion: a young woman from Rhodes, whose family has tourist enterprises in the island, studied psychology and was without work in Athens for years, trying to be appointed to some social welfare centre or in the best case in some psychiatric clinic. Another youth, whose mother has a hotel in Edipsos, a famous spa resort 200 kms north of Athens, studied sociology and, as was to be expected, not being able to find work, had fallen into a vicious circle of low self–esteem, seeing the hopes and dreams of his youth rotting away. However impressive and pompous the sound of a 'degree in sociology' may have seemed to his young ears, as miserable was it to face the stark reality after acquiring it.

And all this waste of youthful spirit of enterprise is caused by parents who do not have the courage to show them the reasonable course to take. They did not want to 'deprive them of the chance to make their dreams come true' they say later, apologetically. However, if something could be imposed on parents to do it would be to transmit their own experience to their children. What they have learned from their own path in life.

Of course I do not mean that the Utopian ideals and actions of young people are worthless, but I do think that just as valuable is the transfusion of wisdom and good sense from the previous generation. It is therefore wrong for parents to have feelings of guilt whenever they try to slow the romantic surges of their children that lead them to make unfounded choices bound to fail. It is my opinion that it is their duty to play their role correctly and wholly comprehensively. And part of a parent's role is also to indicate realistic and applicable life options.

This issue has forcefully come to front stage, precisely because of the financial crisis. As long as there was a boom and things were easy, based on cash being available, it was possible to manage the problems and cover the cracks: a psychologist could find employment in an advertising agency or even be a stylist (those who advise you about what clothes suit your personality!). Today, however, advertising agencies are closing down one after the other and alternative solutions are become rare for the young who invested in hopes and Utopias.

What will happen to all those seeing their dreams vanish? They must either wait for the bullish recovery of the financial cycle, which might be in five or ten years, to begin again from the point they started from, or they will have to reorientate their goals. That is to say, to look around with a fresh approach, free of ideological blinkers, so as to find jobs at which they could <u>work</u>, not 'be occupied'!

Working is not an 'occupation'. It demands effort. And let us not forget that, according to the Old Testament, work is a curse. It was only in Paradise that Man, when first created, did not have to work. He had everything he needed to hand at no cost but outside of that, he was told: "In the sweat of thy face shalt thou eat bread".

The truth is that our generation is so spoil that the notions "work" or "labour" have are progressively became politically incorrect. This distorted signalisation for our young people of the current generation has in essence castrated their competitiveness. They entered the arena of life to enjoy themselves and not to compete. And now, in a time of crisis, they seem disorientated.

Is it our fault, we who were over–protective? Is it due to the course of History, which was overgenerous with them as with no generation before? Whatever the cause, the outcome is that young people today have to take crash courses in competitiveness. The practice of humouring them is coming to an end, as are the parental savings, and pretty soon the resounding and painful 'slaps' will have their turn.

A change as sudden is bound to cause sorrow, anguish and depression. It started out with the men, of about 40 to 60 years old, who were those most exposed to business ventures and loans. The violent redefinition of the economy left them stripped naked, on the one hand as to their working environment and on the other, their family. This because in our society it is more acceptable for a woman to be out of work than a man, upon whose shoulders – whether rightly or wrongly – the burden still remains to sustain the family's financial status.

When the recession set in, I saw executives of companies becoming depressed when they lost their jobs and realised there were no more opportunities for them in similar businesses. I got to know otherwise responsible people who were trying to conceal their dismissal from work from their family. In the face of the dead end before them, they were paralysed. They either waited for a deus ex machina to call them up into a job, or they were so ashamed as well as feeling responsible toward the family, that it came to the point of being stubbornly in denial to face the fact that they were unemployed.

Most suicides belong in this age group. Men who did not only feel useless but, and mainly, that it was their fault. An attempt to minimise their personal responsibility and the shift of the onus onto some general, national, or even better, world–wide crisis frees an individual from the burden of guilt. It gives the crisis a dimension of a generalised war wherein not only individuality is lost but their reflexes operate to protect them personally. A person ceases the self–accusation that leads him into depression and tries instead to protect himself and those he protects – his family dependents – from future worse things to come.

The next victims of the financial crisis appeared in the 30 – 40 age group. In fact in this group the preponderance of men began diminishing. The problem for this group was that they had just begun participating in the party of progress and personal euphoria and were becoming conscious that the festivities were coming to a close. Careers that had just taken off saw their point of support disappearing in the drastic shrinking of their business sector. Personal or familial budgets and plans for life were bursting apart. The worst of all was that there was no sign on the horizon of an easy and accessible solution.

Because of their youth, some made dramatic changes in the orientation of their life: some emigrated, others moved to the provinces. These moves may of course seem somewhat rash in our day but were absolutely normal for foregoing generations. It was also precisely what I urged those who consulted me to do: "All our nation's great benefactors by today's standards were adventurers. The biographies of most of the world's financially successful people are conditional upon their spirit of enterprising business ventures and their being adventurer migrants."

In the present financial crisis, consequently, such people would see the situation as an opportunity instead of a disaster. It forces them to make moves that may in the long run prove to be particularly successful. In the flabbiness of facile prosperity, such moves would have been unthinkable and unimaginable for them.

It meant that people who came to me in the depths of despair went back home to make plans for life's adventures. There is, besides, a fund of dynamic courage harbored by this age group, as of course also in the younger: courage, insolence and love of adventure. These dynamics are suppressed by urban prosperity and the facility inherent in realising the youthful plans for one's life. It is well known that, unfortunately, in the urbanised 'establishment class' love of adventure is usually restricted to the sector of love affairs – frequently extra-marital. The crisis instead offers a real chance to plan and to execute truly adventurous life courses.

As time goes by, the crisis is affecting both extremities of age: the elderly on the one hand, being naturally prone to developing depression, since with the passage of time and life's adversities the serotoninergic circuit of the brain is exhausted, revealing depressive symptomatology. The lack of alternative occupations leads them into the nets of the media's tradition of striking terror with their news bulletins. The bombardment of negative and catastrophic items of news wears out the equivalent mechanism of the brain, resulting in the elderly seeing reality even grimmer and more pessimistic, with no way out. The elderly are less prone to seek psychiatric help, and thus they progressively drown in depression.

For such persons, other than the intake of antidepressants – imperative in these cases – there is the solution of their involvement in organisations and networks of social solidarity. Pensioners can find a new role to play and a purpose in life, coming out of the isolation that comes with old age, through a social activity supervised by local authorities, NGOs, the Church, or other agencies.

Besides, a closer contact of pensioners with social work and real life, places the dimension of the financial crisis on a more correct basis than the exaggerations promoted by the media. It is to be expected and natural, that looming dangers and calamities should be publicised more intensively, since in all animals the instinct of self–preservation makes the antennae more acute and easily stimulated by any threatening signal from the environment. Consequently, worthwhile news is about the approaching threat and not the coming serenity. Therefore, as long as the media are elbowing their way through to top ratings, it is to be expected that they will seek to reveal elements of threat on the horizon and to ignore the rays of light seeping through from the end of the tunnel.

The under thirty–year–olds were the latest victims of the crisis. Initially, the shelter of family care protected them, as did their 'autistic' exclusive preoccupation with their own age group which kept them apart from the actual financial situation. While the economy was disintegrating, they were posting photos on Facebook, sitting–in at their colleges or fighting inside and outside of football fields, to 'defuse' their youthful vitality. When finally they confronted the economic crisis, they believed that their bullying behaviour could oblige the 'bosses' and 'those in charge' to give them back their adolescent dreams which the crisis delays – if not deletes.

In the end, though, this crisis might prove to be a blessing for this age group, because, alas, there was no other way to re–route them in a globalised economy in headlong progressiveness. Their parents were emasculated by the facile conditions of the previous years and incapacitated to show them, by their example, how to become competitive. While, at the same time, the intellectual and political leadership are incapable of generating ideals since in the eyes of the young they are to be disdained for being almost exclusively preoccupied with maintaining their position of power through intrigue and corruption.

Those young people, who come soon to realise that it is useless to await an appointment or a subsidy and make alternative plans for their life, will uncover opportunities for success. Creativity, which comes from the chase and chasing, had unfortunately been weakened by facile economic growth. The financial crisis provides just the motivation our young people needed.

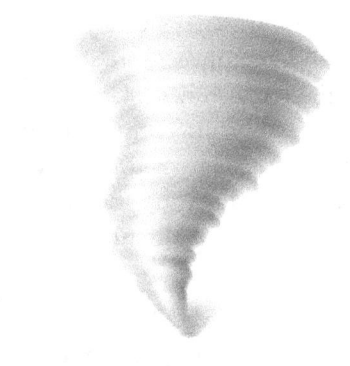

MANIA: A DATA STORM

IT HAS happened to all of us, when surfing the Web; the list of subjects becomes a flood, presented to us by the search engine we employ, of subjects that do not interest us. A classic example is when we have put up a name and surname and the engine gives results corresponding to both. It is natural that this should be confusing. It can also divert our search into fields that have nothing to do with our initial objective. How often will we not in this way have set out on an imprecise ramble, surfing with no direction into sites we had no intention of visiting?

This is exactly what occurs in the symptom that in Clinical Psychiatry we call 'flight of ideas'. The brain's interest in the original subject escapes and certain key words usually lead a manic patient to irrelevant subjects:

— *I saw Victor yesterday... not the French author Victor Hugo... now that I think of it a high school mate of mine lived in Hugo Street... school brings the TV series Play School to my mind...*

When a patient is in a phase of mania their thought process jumps from one subject to another. As a matter of fact, the broadening of the numbers of subjects that the brain is called upon to process impels them to speed the process up. That is what makes it seem as if his mind is racing and processing a series of ideas one after the other, a real flow of ideas. And when the manic patient tries to communicate the flow of ideas flooding the screen of his brain, his speech is unstoppable, he appears to be compelled to keep talking.

I got a phone call that worried me. It was the brother of Elpida, a young woman 28 years old who suffered from depression. She lived in a picturesque spa town and had been brought to me six months earlier by her mother and her brother because when the business where she worked closed and she lost her job, she became depressed. To make matter worse, at the same time as being out of work, Elpida's boyfriend, who worked in the same place, broke up with her. And so Elpida – who her mother told me had always been very active – after being dismissed, not only did not look for another job but stayed indoors at home all the time. She 'sank' so low she didn't even want to watch TV and stayed curled up in bed most of the time.

I prescribed antidepressants for the state she was in and a month later she began going out, seeing people and looking for work. Within two months she had found a job as a sales person and drove around the area in her car. She was apparently taking the antidepressant treatment I prescribed, but she ceased all contact with me.

I should like to say at this point that in the exercise of my profession it is a principle of mine not to initiate a follow up with my patients or their relatives. I don't want anyone to think I am pressing them to come back for another visit. However, in all cases I stress the need, for all my patients as well as their carers, that there has to be psychiatric follow–up, especially when I have prescribed pharmaceutical therapy.

So I didn't know how Elpida was until I received that anguished call from her brother:

– *Doctor, my sister isn't well. She is out half the night, every night, we don't know who she's with and she's out of control from both my mother and from me.*

– *You have to bring her to see me. What is most probable is that she has gone to the other extreme from her depression. I mean, she must be manic.*

– *It won't be easy to bring her. As I said, Doctor, she won't listen.*

– *Tell me something, is she still taking the medication I gave her?*

– *I don't know, I guess not. What I do know is that she's drinking, every day. She often comes home drunk. The worst is we worry that she'll have a fatal accident, the way she drives around.*

– *This is very serious. You have to do something about it. You have to bring her in to be treated. It's your responsibility, yours and your mother's.*

– *But what do you mean? By force?*

— Yes of course by force. The way she is now she doesn't have clear judgement, she doesn't know what she's doing. You can't just let her be and observe discreetly from a distance. You have to do something.

— Well, I don't know. I have to ask my mother…

— Ask what? If you saw her drowning, would you 'ask your mother'? Grab her by the hair and bring her over tomorrow, whenever you can.

I suppose I was so forceful that I convinced him. Next afternoon Elpida came to my office in such a state that I did not recognise her. It was no longer the sweet and modest girl I knew: she had turned into a provocative 'easy lay', with too much make–up and dressed in gaudy colors. Her appearance and her manners were at the limit of vulgarity. She talked stridently and all the time. She would not let anyone put a word in edgewise. If her brother or her mother tried to say something, she interrupted and said loudly:

— I'm here only because the doctor asked me to come. You're too old fashioned and you don't understand me… I shall do as I like and I won't obey anyone. Take it or leave it. Otherwise, I'll leave home and the bird will have flown… Isn't that so, Doctor? I can stay with him. He has a big house and he'll find room for me…

She threw a provocative look – 'meaningful' – in my direction. She was obviously in a manic state, in what in psychiatry we call the manic phase of bipolar disorder, that is, she was manic–depressive. Other than talking all the time, typically, she had also lost self–control.

A week later when she was more balanced she confided in me that in the last ten days she had slept with more than twenty men. She had reached the point of 'coming on' to anyone she saw in front of her. Later, when she had calmed down and was in the phase of full recovery that is, when she could normally resume control of her mood she felt awful and guilty about what she had done while in the manic phase.

It is this remorse about what they have said and done in a manic phase that often brings them to depression. Typically, most of the sufferers have regrets for and feel guilty about their behaviour during the phase. This also serves as an indicator of mania in examination of the patient's history. I ask them if they did things in the past for which they later had regrets.

In bipolar disorder the opposite could also happen. Following a period of depression, an excessive energy may be noticed. Many compare this to the syndrome of the 'chained dog that has been set free', that is to say that after a protracted self–isolation that accompanies depression it is to be expected that the sufferer who is now better should want to go out and have fun. They may even go on a shopping spree.

I remember a patient who came to see me after a year of depression. I gave her the suitable therapy and she came out of her misery. She told me she was enjoying life again at last, going out with her girlfriends and shopping. She said she had been buying all the things she had not bought the whole previous year!

Unfortunately, this understandable 'sub–mania', as it could be called, sometimes notable in curing a depression, often tricks the people around them and their relatives who do not realise in time that the person is entering into a manic phase. The switch can go directly from 'depressed' to 'manic' without their noticing, or being able to judge what are the first indications of mania, so that there may be a delay in starting a pharmaceutical therapy.

So Elpida too, when she became manic tried to flirt with me or, as she put it, to 'come on' to me. In my early years of practice I didn't know how to deal with it and I was embarrassed, but later I learned not only how to handle these admittedly difficult situations but even how to use them to help the patient. A subtle reaction to the flirtatiousness reinforces the therapeutic alliance and the patient is more receptive to medical instructions. There is of course always the risk that the patient will try to cross over the thin red line that keeps the balance and the distance. This is where the practitioner exercises skill to keep the balance, without making so much as a hint of promises, but at the same time not rejecting the patient.

– *Doctor, they said you wanted to see me, so I got all dressed up and here I am…*

– *Let your brother and your mother leave us first, so that you can tell me how you changed.*

Once we were alone together, she saw I was keeping my distance and my purely professional approach. So she restrained her behaviour but she could not hold her tongue. She talked continuously and skipped from one subject to another.

It is noteworthy that even in the most acute phase of either manic or schizophrenic excitation, the patient will adhere to certain codes of communication. They are aware of what they can or cannot do. How far they can go. It is the doctor's role to show the limits for the patient and the limits for the doctor. If the doctor seems relaxed or timid, the patient could exploit this, which would result in eroding, meaning in essence spoiling the therapeutic relationship.

The doctor has to be aware that there is a host of signals transmitted, other than in speech, revealing his or her true intentions. They must consequently be absolutely clear in their mind that they will in no way, compromise their therapeutic relation with the patient. I have to say here that in my career, regrettably, I have come across cases of doctors who have taken advantage of their patients' weakness. 'Doctors' who have taken advantage of loose morals sexually or their patients' financial liberality when they are in a manic phase. I have even heard of 'doctors' who exploited the intellectual weakness and the confusion of mind of schizophrenics, or the diminished judgment of patients with symptoms of senility.

This is how Elpida was now justifying her changed behaviour by claiming the right she had at last, as a woman, to go out and have a good time.

– *Look here, I'm not a little child any more... For years what good did it do me to stay at home, doing what my family wanted me to? Every person has the right, or rather the obligation to do whatever they can, what they are capable of. Me, thank God, I'm beautiful and can arouse men and do what I like with them.*

– *I don't agree. I think on the contrary, that it's the men who think they could take advantage of you, isn't it?*

I always speak in the language close to what my patients use. In that way they feel I am closer to them. They realise I can understand them.

– *Who me? Oh no, nobody can take advantage of Elpida. That man isn't born yet. When he is, I'll tell him. Or rather, you'll be aware of it...*

– *By the stars and the wizards...*

– *Hey, Doctor, don't you mess with me. I'm the star and I'm shining.*

– *But suppose you have been a shining medal on the lapels of some who say they had their way with you and are decorated?*

– *Now, Doctor, that's hurtful.*

– *I'm just telling you the other side of the story which you don't see. I'm not trying to put the brakes on you like your family. Do what you like, be free, but knowing what you're doing.*

It is important for the doctor to dissociate himself from the parents because patients, especially when they are young, nearly always cannot see the doctor in any other role than as their parents' advocate. And additionally, it is the parents themselves who so often place the doctor in that role. It is a classic for parents, when they are trying to control a patient, to say "the doctor said so". But this diminishes the effectiveness of the doctor's advice because it classes the doctor together with the parents, to whose advice the child has already developed 'anti–bodies'.

– *As soon as you asked my parents to wait outside, Doctor, I got it that you are on my side. We two together can do great things. But why are you now being hurtful to me?*

It is typical of patients in mania or just hyper, ('over the top') to be familiar in their speech and actions, such as hugs and kisses, that is when their mood is heightened. This too must be dealt with discreetly. The doctor should not be a buddy but nor rudely reject the advances of friendship by the patient.

— I think you can understand that this euphoria you feel may be lovely, but that it does lead you to act in a way that doesn't compliment you. You take it lightly but other people usually mistake it. I'm afraid that you'll come to regret a lot of what you're doing now…

She was about to interrupt me. In general, talking to manic patients is difficult: they want to talk <u>all</u> the time. Communication is definitely one–sided. Somebody has to cut in otherwise they will not stop talking. In fact for me this characteristic of mania is an aid for my diagnosis. To see if someone is manic I ask them if their interlocutors try to interrupt them. If for instance their friends say: "Please shut up will you? Let us say something too." If this is confirmed, then it means the patient is hypo–manic or manic.

I said:

— Let me say a word or two and then I'll listen to you, for as long as you like. Do you remember that when you were depressed you didn't want to get out of bed, let alone leave the house? Well, now you are at the opposite extreme. Just as that was a pathological state, so is this. As then I helped you regain your energy, now again I must help you get back in control of yourself. The little engine of your brain is turning over too fast and carrying you off course. I can understand that you feel under pressure to talk and do things. You're running in circles and in the end you'll burn out. You have to take medication so that the pace of the brain's engine comes back to normal so that you can control it… It isn't a tranquillizer, don't worry. I'm on <u>your</u> side. I don't want you to be flabby and flaccid. I just want to 'bring you down' a little, one notch. You'll enjoy it more and be better in control, not running after and chasing it.

When you describe what they feel to them they realise you understand them, because however ill they are, they are aware they are in overdrive and cannot control themselves. It is a little like the merry–go–round in the amusement park. They are whirling round and can tell it's potentially dangerous but don't want to get off as they are being told to, because the sensation is exciting and they are enjoying it. In a manic phase patients think they are kings, super–powers. And obviously, it is not a sensation one wants to lose.

As I know how they feel, I propose only a small controlled reduction. Not lose their Paradise, as the 'reasonable' people tell them, nor being 'imprisoned' as their entourage tries to do. What I propose is a third solution: a mild relaxation of the frantic rate so that the course should be controllable by their own self.

Such a proposal is generally acceptable. More so, if I have managed to establish a strong therapeutic alliance with the patient, they will grasp the helping hand I am proffering. They simply do not want to give up that intoxicating sensation. All doctors should try to work with what there is of a healthy part of the thought process. Discreetly, without injuring the disordered part of the patient's existence.

Elpida was persuaded to take lithium. It is not known how this drug affects the brain but we do know it is an effective mood stabiliser. That means it regulates emotions. Not only does it deal with mania, it has been proven that if a bipolar patient is under constant treatment with it, it prevents the reappearance of manic as well as depressive phases, as if it had the switch that turns 'depression' to 'mania' is under control.

One drawback is that unfortunately it does not immediately remedy the mania. A week to ten days is usually required for it to take effect. In many manic cases this is a very long time, because the patient's behaviour has to be put under control immediately. Patients often come to us in a state of frenzy and totally deranged, so that something has to be done right away. Lithium does not bring instant visible moderation. This is why I suggested it to Elpida who I did not want to realise from the start that I was containing her, putting the brakes on her. For instant suppression we use anti–psychotic drugs. These are the drugs used for treatment of schizophrenia.

On the other hand, lithium does not prevent all manic phases but it must be credited, even if it does not prevent them all, that it renders them milder. There are patients who, before commencing lithium treatment went through repeated phases of mania and depression, frequently needing clinical admittance. On lithium prescription, however, decades can go by without a single symptom. Other than lithium – about which it should be noted that it was the first effective psychiatric medication of the past decades, whose performance was confirmed in 1949 – certain anti–epileptic drugs have been found also to have a mood stabilising effect.

The key, however, to the protective action of lithium, as well as the anti–epileptic drugs is in their constant and consistent intake. It has been ascertained that when these drugs are stopped the ups–and–downs of emotions return, and indeed with intensity, and are more difficult to control. Bipolar patients have to realise that if they start a course of lithium or anti–epileptic treatment they have to take it conscientiously and meticulously. Even brief interruptions may not only trigger a fresh access of mania but also an uncontrolled 'to–and–fro' motion of the switch between mania and depression. Of course, as I stressed in the chapter on schizophrenia, the patients themselves are responsible for these developments. They do not abide by the doctors' instructions and very often, when they feel well, try to experiment on their own by ceasing their treatment.

I shall say it once more: it is required of the science of Medicine to make us invulnerable and immortal, but on the other hand we are ready to accuse it of the 'chemistry' and the 'medication' we are saturated with. We accept more easily to wear an amulet all the time than to take our daily medicine. I have known people run to the other end of the world, following the injunctions of their faith, to be cured, instead of following the advice of their doctor. They refuse to stop smoking but cross themselves devoutly in front of every church and crucifix, praying God to keep them well!

To go back to Elpida; I persuaded her to take lithium. Just as I had promised, at first she saw no immediate decrease of the symptoms, so she accepted to continue the treatment. At the same time I told her family to be patient for a few days more and just to make sure that Elpida was taking her medication regularly and keep in touch with me for anything that might occur. Sure enough, a week later they told me she had calmed down a lot and was beginning to be cooperative.

She came back to see me three weeks later. She was much calmer and talked less. She had kept her job despite the side-tracks of the previous period. That was when she confessed her many sexual relations to me. She was beginning to be ashamed of them. It was up to me to relieve her of guilty feelings. I explained that what she had done and said were only the result of her illness. She was not of sound mind, as they say in the law. I told her this to reassure her: that even legally she was exculpated. Nevertheless, she was aware that in her small community the 'legality' did not count: she had been tarnished.

I remember a patient of mine, a married woman, who, in a manic phase had told her husband that she had had an extra-marital affair. I do not know if it was even true or not or if she had said it with the thoughtless superficiality of mania, to show her husband her femininity still counted for something. But the outcome was that I was completely unable to get it out of the husband's head, whatever I said, that she had 'been unfaithful'. It is better not to say things that can't be taken back.

I gathered that Elpida's correct social conduct had gradually restored her reputation in the local community. Not that I think it will be easy for her to find a husband where she lives. But that can be bypassed if she moves to another spot. Sadly, if mania is not soon checked it is usually a serious stigma on the sufferer. They are helplessly exposed to acting in a way that cannot be concealed in the 'town crowd' and are neither easily forgiven nor forgotten.

Whereas depression is a torment for the sick person themselves, mania on the contrary mainly makes for problems with the person's entourage. In depression it is the sick person who suffers, in mania it is those around them. In many cases the family of a bipolar patient is better off when the patient is in a depressive phase and even dreads that a normal mood state could suddenly precipitate their sick relative to mania.

The truth is that a sufferer of mania can be extremely tiresome. They talk a lot, their voice is strident, they roam around all the time, they are hyper-active. They are besides possessed by an excessive optimism so that they shop extravagantly or undertake high-risk business ventures. If they are on the whole intelligent and have some good luck such moves may benefit them. In this way some bipolar patients are successful business persons but, there are others who bring about enormous financial disasters both for themselves as for their entourage.

Hypomania

IT IS THEREFORE easy to understand that the crux of the matter is the 'extent' of the mania. If the sufferer exceeds some limit and loses touch with reality, the next step is easily a sort of delirium: "*I am a divinity... I am invulnerable... I can govern the world... I am wealthy.*" When they reach that stage of psychotic condition, they lose their judgment, their control of reality and of course those they come into contact with will censure them.

If, however, they are kept at a level of mere super-optimism then the risks they usually take may lead to some success. In the 80s there was a merchant who had the bright idea of selling consumer products to be paid for in installments by civil servants. He saturated Athens with advertisements. Things apparently went well at first. He opened branches in various neighbourhoods. But, alas, a year later his family brought him to be sectioned in my psychiatric clinic, in a totally manic state. His initial profits pushed him to place unrealistic orders for goods he could not sell. He began lowering prices to considerably under their purchase cost. His mania did not allow him to think reasonably. If anyone warned him that he was heading for disaster he would compare himself to major retail sales chain stores where some products are sold below cost price. He would not listen to anybody. As was to be expected, he went bankrupt, but continued blaming his family who did not share his optimism as to his prospects and refused to lend him capital sums.

The combination for success

I believe that the best mixture to ensure a person's success is:

- To be intelligent
- To be hysterical
- To be in a constant state of hypomania

Hypomania helps one to be slightly more optimistic than the 'normal' average and to take more risks. Who risks nothing, gains nothing. Had there never been some 'crazy guy' to leave his cave and build a shelter with sticks, man would still be living in caves. A degree of overestimation of one's potential is necessary in order to step out to actions that might lead to success otherwise one will stay put and not attempt any improvement.

Hypomania is also of assistance in increasing one's dynamism beyond the norm. Thought processes operate faster and more ideas are produced in the brain. It is as if they had a quicker processor and a search engine with expanded filters. Thus, ideas abutting the central subject enter the framework of the processing.

If, besides a degree of mania, a person also has a degree of intelligence, it is possible for the combination of new ideas to bear fruit and lead to success. Great inventors were occupied with a variety of activities, their attention was not focused on a single objective.

Finally, I shall develop in another chapter an analysis of the hysterical characteristics of a personality required to be successful. I mention here only that in psychiatry we say a person is hysterical when they want to be the centre of attention. A hysterical person handles emotion masterfully and thereby communicates better. In that way they can be more persuasive with those around them and consequently have better chances of success in life.

Therefore, since a level of hypomania is desirable in most bipolar patients, the psychiatrist often finds him or herself in a crossfire. The family wants the sufferer as much as possible under control, i.e. 'low' or just at the limit of depression. The patient on the other hand wants to be as 'high' as possible.

This is where the psychiatrist enters the picture with his medication. His role is that of a theatrical director, or rather a team coach. He monitors developments and regulates, ever with the supreme criterion in mind of the patient's best interest.

In my career I have often felt I was playing with fire. I submitted to a patient's pressures but feared the sudden resurgence of mania, which would create bigger problems. An expert knowledge of pharmacology is needed and, especially, serious cooperation with both the sufferer and their entourage.

It needs to be observed when the sufferer begins to sleep less. When they talk more and will not be interrupted. When they do more extravagant shopping. These three elements: insomnia, to be more talkative than usual, and over–consumerism are the corner–stones of mania, immediately noticeable. The appearance of one of those has to galvanise their carers to contact the doctor right away.

I talk about such things with the patients themselves, in the presence of those who accompany them, so as to attain a degree of therapeutic alliance three ways: with the sick person, their entourage and the doctor. When those three sides of the triangle function in cooperation then, and only then, will the bipolar patient be safe.

As an extreme instance I frequently refer to a politician who was bipolar.

As long as the three sides worked together efficiently, his treating psychiatrist maintained him at all times in a hypomanic state, with the most positive results for the Party and the country. However, when after a certain point his close partners refused to control him, the equilibrium was disturbed. They did not exert sufficient pressure on him, when he began to tend towards mania. They even let him stop his treatment. The outcome was not only that he brought ridicule upon himself but, what was much worse, that the national institutions were debased to an unprecedented degree, so that naturally corruption flourished and of course brought about his country's financial ruin.

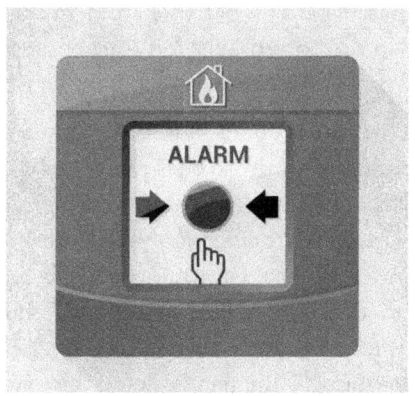

ANXIETY AND PANIC ATTACKS: A USELESS ALARM SYSTEM

Anxiety's prehistory

THE FIRST time I heard it, it made a great impression on me. The word anxiety is in essence an invention of the twentieth century. Earlier, human beings were not only free of anxiety but did not even have a word for what is so generalised in our day. It is probable that Freud first used the German 'Angst' in this sense. He will have been inspired by the ancient Greek term 'αγχόνη' (ankhoni) meaning 'gallows' that is, pressing the neck. It later came into English as 'anxiety' and returned to Greek as 'άγχος' (ankhos).

Although, as I learned later, of course already in Antiquity Hippocrates had described the symptom as 'pnix' from the word 'to choke', it is nevertheless a fact that the general adoption of the Freudian theories is related to the increased frequency of appearance of 'anxiety' in the West at the dawn of the twentieth century. So it was inevitable that the term employed by Freud should have been generalised all over the world for that symptom.

When, therefore, at the end of the nineteenth century and beginning of the twentieth, cases began to appear – they were mostly women – with a pronounced symptom of a 'knot in the throat', psychiatrists of those days called it the 'hysterical knot', from the Greek hysterikos (= of the womb). What was then called hysteria is none other than what we now call anxiety.

The most frequent manifestation of hysteria at the beginning of the twentieth century was hysterical paralysis. The patients suddenly felt they could not move their legs or an arm. Also they often believed they could not feel that limb at all. Sometimes they felt no pain, even when pricked with a needle.

It should of course be remembered that in the nineteenth century in Europe people were afraid of paralysis. In those days polio and other contagious diseases of the nervous system wrought havoc, so it is understandable that women between the ages of 20 to 40 were afraid of being paralysed. This is why anxiety manifested itself as paralysis. When the mechanism of over–vigilance was activated and the young woman went into what today we call a panic, she suddenly thought she could not walk, or not move her arm. And as is the case today too in a state of panic, the disturbing sensation of the paralysis fed the over–alertness in a cycle of positive feedback i.e. self–re–supply.

In the Western world today there are no longer cases of hysterical paralysis. The last one I remember in my career was when I was resident in neurology. It was a beautiful girl from Crete named Maria who, due to family problems, after a quarrel with her mother–in–law, suddenly could not get out of bed. That was the case history initially given us by the relatives who brought her to the hospital. Both her legs were paralysed. The symptom was quite serious and worrying. They therefore brought her to Athens, to the university neurological clinic, fearing a serious neurological illness.

In spite of her evident disability, the young patient seemed impassive and calm, what in the old days psychiatrists called "belle indifference" – beautiful indifference. Obviously, her disability had a beneficial effect on the girl. All the concern shown by her relations had helped her out of her psychological difficulties. As I ascertained from her later case–history, in essence her disability protected her from her in–laws' criticisms.

When I had comforted her as to her paralysis and reassured her that the condition was reversible, I tried to show her that on the one hand I could understand the problems tormenting her and on the other, mainly, that I would not be critical of her. It goes without saying that I promised her total confidentiality, and I asked her to open her heart to me. I also gave her an anti–anxiety injection, to lower the level of her stress, to relax her and to 'loosen her tongue'. An anti–anxiety medicine acts like alcohol. It brings about a slight suspension of inhibitions. We know that under the influence of alcohol most of us have revealed things that would normally not pass our lips.

Half an hour later, when she was reassured that I was her ally, her unconcerned manner gave way to loud sobs. From the bottom of her heart she confessed that although she was newly married, when she went to market she felt it beating for a man from her village. She felt guilty because of her social inhibitions. Particularly when the man realised she was attracted and reciprocated the burning glances. She was ashamed and quickly went home. There, she thought her mother–in–law saw from her face – probably blushing – that there was something improper going on, and when the older woman asked what the matter was, she went straight to bed. Unfortunately for her, in the marital bed her thoughts of the other man flamed, but at the same time so did her guilty feelings and consequently the anguish. The mother–in–law came into the bedroom, and asked more anxiously, and perhaps with more severity, what had happened. The young woman did not answer and the other became even more strict, telling her to get out of bed quickly and go and do her household chores. Maria then tried to get up and found she could not stand. She tried to move, and fell over flat in front of the bed.

— *She shouted at me to stand up and then I realised my legs did not obey me. I panicked. I thought I was paralysed. Or rather, that God had paralysed my legs for me never to leave the house and meet this other man. God was punishing me but at the same time protecting me.*

Sobbing, the girl told me all. I answered that her emotions were absolutely justified and that all of us had felt them too.

— *Your husband himself might think about another woman in the same way. It isn't a crime. It doesn't mean it's a catastrophe to be attracted to somebody that one shouldn't.*

I went on talking to her soothingly in this sense, holding her hand. I let her speak and was acquitting her of guilt.

— *I'm quite sure your mother–in–law's heart too will have beaten for someone other than your father–in–law.*

I said it laughing. She smiled, she squeezed my hand and tried to move her legs.

— *Don't be in a rush, my dear. As I promised, you'll not only be able to stand, you'll be dancing.*

A doctor has to be able to contain his enthusiasm. He has to be confident of his therapy and in what he does but not fall into the trap of being enthusiastic over some minor subjective improvements, most of which are temporary. He must be wary of rejoicing too soon, as it is so often followed by disappointment.

— *You've been under a great deal of stress and you need to rest. Your legs will gradually start functioning again. The wonder–working injection I gave you helped. But don't rush it and don't be upset if you're not back to normal straight away.*

In his relation to a patient a doctor must at all times exercise restraint, because if the patient realises his or her heightened anticipation they may disappoint them on purpose, the only reason to cast doubt on their 'omnipotence', just as we did at school when we liked to 'pin down' a teacher. There is always a difficult game being played between patient and doctor. That is where the practitioner's skill lies: to change the game played where there is a victor and a loser, to one where both are winners. There are in my experience many pitfalls in this process that can at any moment entirely overturn the whole therapeutic effort. That however is the great charm of medical talent as well as of its technique!

In the ensuing years I came across some instances of hysterical amnesia. Memory loss is another nightmare recently appeared to haunt our Westernised society. The more society transited from manual labour to an economy based on the workings of the mind and the 'services rendered' by the brain, the more a person's anxieties were transferred from paralysis to amnesia. One heard of someone having a stroke and afterwards not being able to speak or read. Other patients, after a stroke, had only lapses of memory. These symptoms seemed strange, uncanny, and, of course peculiarly threatening to many of us, especially those whose work depends on their mental capacities.

I once saw a young ship's captain who came back home after many months at sea, and somebody told him his young bride had been unfaithful. From the same evening he began to be unable to remember anything. The shock evidently not only led him to block the distressing fact but everything else as well. He could not remember who he was nor his name, his address, his relatives and friends. He was in a daze, like a stranger who knew nothing about his familiar surroundings. Everything appeared to him as seen for the first time.

When I examined him I saw that not only could he remember everything from that moment on but he also had memories of many things from the past, just as long as they had nothing to do with the people around him. He could, for example, describe in detail scenes from his military service but did not remember if he was married and who his friends were! His relatives seemed to be more anguished than he was himself. Typically, he kept saying:

– *They tell me I'm married to that girl but I don't remember anything…*

When his family members brought the seaman to the clinic I knew nothing about his wife's affair. I suspected something, but none of the relatives wanted to say anything about it. He himself could, of course, not give any information, since he was amnesiac. I reassured him and the people close to him too.

With a little anxiety–relieving medication, no pressure at all and lots of patience, in a few hours the patient 'blabbed'. A psychiatrist, you see, has not only to be well informed of the cultural conditions of the patient's surroundings but very often also has to be a detective. He must have the nose of a sleuth and sniff out where the problem lies. So, I took the conversation to more sensitive areas where I thought the source of his anxiety lay. At the same time I was careful to eliminate the emotional charge the people with him had for the sufferer.

— *In those various ports, when you went ashore you frequented some women, didn't you?*

— *Mmm... It sometimes happens... It's nothing special.*

— *Yes, I know, some trifling relationship with no follow-up...*

— *Exactly, no follow-up*

— *And it's no crime, is it, Captain?*

— *Of course not.*

— *Besides, it does no harm to anyone. Not to your wife, nor the children.*

— *Weeell, I don't know...*

— *It doesn't harm your wife if you go with another woman... It's not as if you were going to leave her for someone else, is it?*

— *That's right, it's nothing bad for her.*

— *Nothing bad will happen to me either, Captain, if as we speak my wife goes with another man. As long as she doesn't lose her head and wants to leave me. What do I care what she does when I'm not with her! I could be with a babe right now, instead of being with you. If it doesn't threaten the harmony of our marriage, there's no problem. Am I right, Captain?*

— *It isn't that easy, old boy. How can you dismiss everything? If you go on like that, you and your wife will break up very soon.*

— *I guess you're right, Captain. But if it only happens once it's no crime.*

— *No, one slip isn't the end of the world.*

— *So it isn't the end of the world for you either, is it? Nothing will happen to you if in all those months you've been away your wife went with another man once. Going astray once doesn't matter, isn't that so?*

— *Doctor, now you're making it difficult for me.*

— *If she's o.k. in everything else... Is she to be condemned for one little fault? Come on! Where are we living? It isn't as if it's a rare thing to happen. I don't think there's a single man, or woman for that matter, who hasn't gone astray at some time. Whether it was serious or not, as long as it's over. In fact I can tell you from my experience that sometimes it even reinforces the relationship...*

— *Yeah, next you'll be telling me it's a good thing.*

— *Why not? You know what I mean, it arouses the blood and the mind...*

— *Wow, Doctor, how very advanced you are!*

These favourite tactics of mine, of striking at the sensitive spot while at the same time making light of the distress or, as they say, 'blowing hot and cold', bring the patient to the point of relaxation in confronting what he feared and thought to be disastrous. Of course, I had also administered an antidepressant with an anti–anxiety drug. So, a few hours later, the patient began to 'remember'.

I saw him again in a few days. He was no longer stressed, and his depression when he learned of his wife's infidelity was not a threat to him anymore. His emotional state gradually improved and he started seeing things from a more optimistic angle.

I met his wife and told her emphatically on no account to make the mistake of owning up to anything, and most of all never to answer demands to give details. It is better that such subjects should not be given precision and they stay nebulous, between reality and fantasy.

This is the way, if the companion goes along with it, for the injured party to come to 'forget' in the future or to resort to the mechanism of 'denial'. I have known lots of people, of both sexes, who after a short while blocked out the fact of the infidelity, or found psychological 'comfort' in attributing it all to others' wickedness!

If on the contrary the infidelity is officially labelled, imagination gnaws at the daily trivia: "What was he like? Was he better in bed? Where did you do it? How did you do it? What did he say to you?" All this and much more that cannot be foreseen because imagination has no limits may be dancing around in the mind of the other partner, which results in the poisoning of the couple's relationship for good. This is why I say again and again that couples should never indulge in true confessions, unless they have decided to end the relationship.

When the captain was again in good spirits a few weeks later, I said goodbye with these words:

— *Life is a very interesting journey. Inevitably it has its storms, but remember, whoever survives bad weather will enjoy the calm. After the storm there is always fine weather. We must focus always on the good times to come.*

Modern anxiety

BY NOW, today, the meaning of the word 'anxiety' is no longer exclusively connected to being 'throttled'. It has taken on a more general sense covering the spectrum of hysterical paralysis to the plague of the times, which is hypochondriac ideations and panic attacks. In hypochondria the patient interprets the diverse 'innocuous' physical symptoms they have as the symptoms of a malignant disease, whereas in a panic attack they are more afraid of sudden death from a heart attack or a stroke. In our modern society, you see, patients manifest their anxiety in whatever people fear most in our Western post–industrial society: death from cancer or sudden death from a cardio–vascular disease.

The term 'hypochondria' derives from the two anatomical parts below the ribs where the spleen is on the left side and the liver on the right. These are the spots where most of these patients feel pain or general discomfort.

However, mind you, this discomfort is not in their imagination, but what they feel comes from malfunction of their organs and not from any anatomical deformation of them. That is to say it is not that the organs have something wrong with them – a tumour for instance – but that in most cases there is hyper–functioning because of rising number of signals from the brain.

For when the brain is over–active it signals to the organs to go into 'over–drive'. The heart will beat faster or breathing will be more rapid, or the gastro–intestinal tube will have intensified peristalsis and spasms or excessive excretion of gastric fluids. It is understandable that all bodily functions are controlled by the brain. That is usually where the dysfunction exists.

However, most of these persons are afraid that the fault is in their peripheral organs, that there is damage to their heart or their intestine. This scares them and, as is to be expected, the anxiety increases the stress and consequently generates even greater disturbance in the peripheral organs. This becomes a vicious circle, increasing the alertness and over–functioning, and frequently the patients have the strong conviction that they have some malignant disease of the organ that is simply over–functioning.

Never shall I forget a pretty 30–year–old woman who, when she came to see me, had her hair cut so short it was almost shaven. I thought at first it was the fashion and did not comment on it. She had come to me because she was very anxious, fearing she had cancer. She had stomach aches and frequent diarrhoea. The pain would appear in different places, accompanied by rumbling. She was certain it was cancer but avoided having the necessary tests, being afraid of the results.

So sure was she, not only of the diagnosis – she had looked it up on the Internet, so she 'knew'— she was also certain of the treatment she would be prescribed or recommended: chemotherapy, which would cause her hair to fall out. Therefore, she had taken one step ahead and cut her hair off!

Just imagine the degree of anxiety that these unfortunates reach. In essence, it ruins their life, it cripples them grievously. Everybody should be aware of it: anxiety is a serious illness requiring a serious response.

The words I often hear, unfortunately also from colleagues, are *"Well, you are stressed… It's nothing."* The epitome of superficiality! It is the worst advice anybody can give to someone who is suffering. While they are suffering, you show either that you are mocking them or that you do not believe what they claim.

The mechanism of anxiety

ANXIETY MAY be considered a state of excessive alertness of the organism. It is a reaction of the organism to external threatening stimuli. The reaction enables a person to confront the threatening stimulus or to distance them from it (the well-known fight or fly reaction).

The sight of a dangerous animal, for example, may provoke tachycardia, meaning that the flow of blood to the heart is increased. This is a reaction controlled by the autonomous nervous system, which at the same time directs the blood where it is most needed, i.e. to the muscles. They will be more effective with a greater supply of blood, either to fight the animal or to escape from it. Even a red face or raised hairs on the body – usually brought on by fear – are the primordial reactions that make a person seem more threatening to the opponent. It is the same as in cats whose fur 'stands on end' when they are under threat so as to look bigger and more savage.

Sweating is nothing more than preparation of the organism for a potential increase in body temperature, expected to occur from running away or from muscular exertion of fighting the animal.

It can therefore be seen that these reactions are a primitive, primal programming, provoked in a being almost automatically, without any particular thought and logical data processing. It is obvious that it helped a very speedy preparation of the organism either to fight the opponent or get away fast. It is reasonable thought that presses the alarm button, immediately and automatically provoking this autonomous reaction. It means that when an animal senses danger, it gives the instructions to the autonomous nervous system instantly to prepare the organism either to fly or fight.

The alarm is activated by simply 'pressing a button', like a trigger. It is not equipped with a 'rheostat' so that the intensity of reaction may be progressively regulated, as for instance we increase the sound of a loudspeaker. And this is so because, if it were gradually progressive, it would not have immediate effect. In the case that the alarm had an intermediary 'rheostat', until the victim decided how much the heartbeats should be increased to augment cardiac function and if it should sweat or go red in the face or not, it would probably already have been devoured.

Control of the Anxiety

– It all started four years ago, Doctor, on the 25th of July. It was a very hot day and I was in a hurry to do some errands before going away on holiday. I went to the tax office. The lift wasn't coming so I decided to take the stairs. Just before I reached the first floor my heart started beating furiously. I slowed down a bit but got there, although I was out of breath. There was a crowd and the atmosphere was unpleasant. For a second a thought went through my mind: "Suppose I faint, what a to–do there will be!" But instead of calming down, my heart beat even faster… I felt extremely unwell and all I wanted to do was to get out of the building… I turned around and took flight as if I was escaping something. Outside, I took deep breaths… I still remember it, it was a nightmare. Ever since, whenever my heart beats faster, I am paralysed.

From the moment the alarm goes off, that is when the signal of a stressful reaction is given, the situation is not controlled by logic. This means that our thoughts cannot regulate the degree of heartbeats provoked by a given reaction.

A significant factor making the autonomous alert a pathological state is the sensation of malaise it brings a person. In this way, subjective discomfort, perhaps from an excessive reaction of the heart for instance, depends on three things:

Firstly, on the extent of the reaction that was provoked, that is how many heartbeats to the minute. We should know that the alarm going off does not produce the same rate in all people. For some it may reach 80 and in others 120.

Second, on the condition of the targeted organ – in this case the heart. If, however, as happens in many people, there is a problem in the heart's pacemaker, this escalation of frequency may bring about extra contractions. This of itself will cause a negative feeling and will discomfort the subject. I must emphasise here that these problems of cardiac conductivity in most cases do not usually require special treatment. They present only when the alarm bell rings. Thus, the treatment indicated is consequently prevention of unnecessary alarms.

Thirdly, on the readiness of the mind to be conscious of any anomaly in the function of the heart. When we are calm, none of us is conscious of our heart's function. We are so only when we 'pant'. There must be some filter which below some level does not inform us of the rate of our heart–beat. That regulates itself with an auto–regulating mechanism. Thus, when we climb stairs the heart beats faster, again without our noticing it as something out of the ordinary. The function regulates itself so as to supply the increased blood flow where it is needed without our being warned. Only when the pulse exceeds some limit that the filter of our logical thought – let's say our judgment – has set, then our cerebral cortex becomes aware that there is something going on and is called in to intervene. Alerting the cortex has the purpose of telling the organism "watch what you are doing, because your pulse is racing and you don't have much leeway." In the same way the hunted animal decides to hide or fight, since it cannot run any faster.

Therefore, after an episode of tachycardia, modern Man, who has heard about cardiac arrest and is more afraid of it than anything else, sets the level of the notification filter at a lower cardiac frequency. In this way, even at a pulse rate of 85 or 95, the cortex receives the danger signal. The phenomenon is often seen of the cortex being notified sooner than is the norm. So, of course, in turn it lowers the 'alert limit' even more, resulting in the vicious circle leading to the subjectively extremely unpleasant state of a panic attack.

This means that a fortuitous tachycardia may provoke a feeling of cardiac indisposition which will in turn bring about the feeling of fear and consequently an anxiety reaction. This recycling of anxiety sometimes leads to manifestation of panic, to the extent of what is called a 'premonition of imminent death'.

The usefulness of anxiety

IT IS A FACT that small quantities of anxiety are productive and belong to human beings' adaptation mechanisms. It keeps the organism in a state of vigilance, ready to deal with dangers and adverse circumstances of the environment. In our day of course, situations of danger do not arise from wild beasts and do not usually have anything to do with physical fighting or flight. Tachycardia and an increased blood flow to the muscles are consequently absolutely superfluous physical reactions. The same goes for raising hair, perspiration, redness of face, that is, blushing. Actually, not only are they superfluous, they can also make us ridiculous in the eyes of those around us. Who of us does not feel embarrassed when we know we are blushing or sweating? Particularly if our reaction is noticeable by others.

Furthermore, reactions of the gastro–intestinal system are not only superfluous, they are harmful, such as stomach spasms and intensive intestinal activity that can lead to vomiting, diarrhoea or what is known as spastic colitis. So are reactions of the urinary tract such as frequent urination, as well as of the breathing apparatus, panting and laryngeal muscle spasm that sometimes give a sensation of choking.

I shall always remember the first time I asked to speak at a psychiatric conference when I was a fresh psychiatric resident. When I was handed the microphone, I could not utter a word. My throat had closed and the first sound I was able to make was a croak, while my face was bright red and I was dripping with sweat.

All these reactions could at some time have helped a human and his generic predecessors to confront dangers of their surroundings. Nowadays however these automatic reactions can cause only problems for modern Man.

Exceptional situations of danger do not require muscular effort in our days. They usually require a decision and not only a swift one but often also a difficult one. Today a human being is constantly on the horns of a dilemma that has to be solved by the mind and not the body.

A physical alarm system is in consequence unnecessary and may even often distract the person's attention from the real problem as it provokes physical discomfort. This discomfort frequently triggers questioning and thoughts of possible health problems. In such a process many people are led to manifest hypochondriac fears and symptoms. This creates a chronic source of anxiety resulting in constant hyper–activity of the autonomous nervous system.

The impact of anxiety

CHRONIC EXPOSURE of the organism to anxiety naturally causes wear and tear. A heart that is always functioning at high frequency without performing a particular functional purpose is to be expected to present problems earlier that it should. The same applies to the other organs controlled by the autonomous nervous system. Blood pressure climbs without being able to be relieved by a muscular exercise such as would occur normally in a reaction of fight or flight. Purposeless whipping of specific organs will naturally in the long run provoke deterioration both in the vessels and the organs they supply.

It may therefore be concluded that chronic anxiety is deleterious not only for the mental but also for one's physical health. All our organism's systems are affected, from the circulation to the urinary–genital.

Stress produces frequent urinary output as well as sexual impotence. For men in particular the effect of anxiety or any mental pressure is devastating. The rumour is well known that circulated in the army among recruits that some substance was added to the drinking water which reduced their sexual ardour. It is, of course, more probable that it was the stress they were under that brought impotence rather than any conspiratorial ingredient, a figment of their imagination.

Besides, here the observation of many women is apt, that the best lover is the mindless lover, or as some women say, a 'carefree' lover. Men and women should know that the more a man tries to satisfy a woman sexually and the more anxious he feels about it, the worse his performance will be. Sexologists call this the 'performance anxiety'.

It is similar to an actor who, the more anxious he is when performing, the more mistakes he will make. This is why even veteran actors will have a shot of whisky before a performance to reduce their anxiety. It calms them down and they come on stage relaxed. Just as long as they do not overdo it and stagger on to the stage! The same thing happens with some nervous prospective lovers. They have such a lot to drink so as to relax that all they do when they reach bed is go to sleep.

Women are lucky in that they do not have the same problem. If they wish, they are capable of shamming satisfaction, even that they reached orgasm. And if the signs of orgasm may be recognised by one who knows something about it, I don't think his pride would let him admit he was 'fooled' by his companion who has gone to the trouble to pretend so as to please him!

A piece of advice

CONSTANT ANXIETY, as has been said, is bad for the organism. A frightened brain whips the body to be more efficient. It is like driving a car in second gear and high rpms. It is to be expected that the engine will tire, heat up, and that its output will fail earlier than designed by the manufacturer than if it had had a normal or gentle treatment.

So, I often tell my patients to relax. Go into fourth gear or even higher. Wind the window down and put your arm out of it. Enjoy the drive... Notice how pleasant it is... And more importantly, look at the seat beside you. If someone is sitting next to you, see that they have a good time and know that if they are happy you too will be better off. Happiness is contagious, just as grumbling is.

If they can drive, pull over and ask to change places. That will give you a rest and increase that person's self–confidence. Remember always that what counts is not how fast you will reach your destination but how you are when you get there, in what frame of mind and with what impressions you have garnered from the trip. What counts is the journey to Ithaca, as the poet says. Not merely the speed. Think that if Odysseus had reached home straight away, we would not be speaking of the Odyssey today. Homer would have written some couplet that would have been forgotten!

So take the place of the co–driver, even for a short while. Sit comfortably, relaxed, sprawl in the seat. Show the driver you trust them, at least as much as you would wish them to trust you. Don't bother with the driving but what you are traversing. Look around you, now you aren't driving, you can do it. And something else, look behind you at the back seat. There could be children there you did not pay attention to. Laugh with them and say something about the trip. They need to learn from your experience.

The relation between anxiety and depression

AS HAS BEEN said, anxiety is due to hyper–alertness, to excessive excitation of some neural circuits in the brain. GABA (gamma–aminobutyric acid) is an endogenous substance reducing the excitation of neural cells. If therefore a medicine is prescribed that imitates GABA it will result in containment of the excitation and consequently of the anxiety. Such drugs are the well–known anxiolytic or tranquilizing preparations. A similar effect is achieved with alcohol, mankind's earliest sedative i.e. anxiolytic medication invented.

It has however been observed that anxiolytic drugs are not the definitive solution to anxiety by themselves. They will temporarily reduce the anxiety but evidently cannot cure the causes of it. Scrutinising the case history of patients having panic attacks or other manifestations of anxiety, it will be seen that it all began when the person was having a hard time psychologically. Anxiety reveals itself and spreads when there is mental strain, which is known to produce stress in the serotonin and adrenaline circuits responsible for depression.

It has been observed on the other hand, that if the anxiety is not treated and becomes chronic, the sufferer may show signs of depression. This not due only to the disability entailed by anxiety when it is an everyday condition but it is evident that there is some common pathophysiology in both anxiety and depression.

Specialists are now convinced that to combat anxiety radically, antidepressant treatment is also required, reinforcing the serotonin and adrenaline circuits, to exert an indirect effect on the vulnerability for revealing up–surging anxiety. Let us say they hamper the easy pressing of the 'alarm button'. It seems that when the neuronal circuits of depression are unable to operate successfully they lose control of the 'alarm' that can then be activated more easily and for no serious reason.

It is also commonly observed that the existence of anxiety, often accompanied by depression, provokes a deterioration of physical symptoms, whether objectively or subjectively. The best clients of general practitioners and cardiologists are patients suffering from anxiety. It is nevertheless noteworthy that colleagues of those specialisations seem inefficient in dealing with them, knowing from experience that they will not be able to satisfy them. An anxious patient coming out of the cardiologist's office carrying a normal ECG and the doctor's assurance that 'there is nothing wrong with the heart' is not satisfied. The doctor's reassurance leaves them dissatisfied, because they know the symptoms will recur.

They are, besides, also exposed to those who accompanied them to the doctor, because it appears that they underwent the whole procedure for no good reason. A patient who has crises of anxiety with physical symptoms would really prefer the doctor to have diagnosed something serious. In fact, if we think that it is usually a case of emergency admittance to hospital, the disappointment of the patient and those who accompany him may be imagined when the doctors tell them the patient has no pathological problem.

The next time, because there is always another anxiety attack, the relatives look at the patient reproachfully, as if to say: "oh no, not again!" Because of course, everybody knows at that moment that the alarm is phony. It is literally what is occurring; a false alarm from the sufferer's brain. Not consciously, because the person suffering the most is the patient himself.

I had a patient who could not leave Athens because it was only in the capital with its numerous hospitals that she felt safe. She had a map in her mind, in fact, of the location of the hospitals so as to know at all times which one was closest. She believed she could not leave the periphery of the city. She had never been on holiday in the five years she suffered from anxiety attacks. In essence she was living in a prison. She realised it was unreasonable but, as for most persons in this category, she thought that she was 'eccentric', a condition she could not get over, like a bad habit that cannot be stopped.

The fault is in the attitude of our society, that anxiety is something we can control by ourselves. So these patients feel they are weak, just as they consider their ailment to be a weakness of theirs. This is why most of them try to conceal it and are reluctant to ask for help. I think we are duty bound to speak out about this grave misunderstanding that condemns uncounted persons to live imprisoned in this illness.

An ex–student of mine asked me to help her shortly after she graduated. She had been posted to a provincial community clinic in an Ionian Island. She moved to the island with the help of her parents, drove them back to Athens and now had to go back alone to take up her duties.

She was asking for my help because she was desperate about her condition. She confided in me that on the trip out from Athens she had noted the emplacement of every hospital and health centre along the way, as well as of the time needed to get from one spot to the other. Her mind had rehearsed the scenario of the route Athens to the port of Patras and from there to the island. "A quarter of an hour out of Athens I'll be near the Elefsina's hospital. From there, if I put on speed, in 25 minutes I'll be near Corinth where there is a big hospital. I have calculated the time needed from there to every next hospital in Aigion and Patras. I'll be speeding, driving with clenched teeth."

Another patient confided to me that she never went to venues that were closed. She would try to persuade her companions not to go to cinemas, nor the bigger entertainment centres. She would think up a new excuse, either that it was not a good film or that she had a headache or that she had heard about a new restaurant. And when she did go out somewhere she would find a seat close to an exit. She preferred a table near the door. If after all she couldn't avoid the cinema she always sat at the outside end of the row, preferably at the back, near the exit.

When I had treated this young woman and she was well, she rang me up one Sunday lunchtime to tell me joyfully that the evening before she had gone to a noisy nightclub with a live show and that she had been sitting at a table right in front of the stage. She also said, full of pride as well as gratitude, that she had chosen the seat closest to the stage. It was where it is most difficult to get away fast and where the whole room could see her!

There are innumerable cases of 'imprisoned' people who either do not seek help or go to a general physician, cardiologist, gastroenterologist, lung specialist, urologist or any other specialisation than a psychiatrist. And of course, if after the examination the GP or cardiologist should recommend – which rarely happens – a visit to a psychiatrist, the patient will assume either that he is not believed or that they are rejected by the doctor. It often happens that they will answer:

– Why are you sending me to a psychiatrist? Don't you believe me? Do you think I'm crazy? That I imagine things? Didn't you see my pulse is racing and how high my blood pressure is? Do you think my coming to see you is a joke? You think I want to waste my time and my family's?

A doctor's proper reply should be:

– Of course not. I just think your problem is not cardiovascular but that it's in your brain. You have a specific fault in the brain that is better dealt with by a psychiatrist.

In this way the patient will not feel rejection and will go to a psychiatrist just as they would go to an urologist if the GP had said the problem was urological. But sadly what usually happens is disastrous. Usually, the general practitioner, cardiologist or gastroenterologist, after sending the patient to have all sorts of tests, useful or useless, will pat them on the back and say there's nothing wrong with them. Or, if the patient insists, will prescribe an anxiolytic drug, not only telling them to take as little as possible of it but, warning them against making too much use of it, because "these medicines are habit–forming". This attitude of a doctor can only be called disastrous.

Furthermore, being sent to have tests really only reinforces the anxious patient's hypochondriac conviction that they have some physical illness. A particularly serious one, moreover, since the doctor has told them to undergo serious – and especially, expensive – tests. Also, the recommendations for an anxiolytic sedative treatment, given in the way they are, are generally not effective. This is because when there is an 'attack', the anxiety comes to a peak and a minimal dose of sedative drug cannot deal with it. And what's more, this tactic of 'minimal anxiolytic treatment' often leads the patient to believe that the symptoms are not due to stress, since the drugs cannot control them. Finally, the attitude of most doctors who are not specialists and do not know enough about anxiolytics, discredit these beneficial drugs patients are in such need of.

The treatment for anxiety in five steps

1. THE FIRST step to win the patient over is to show that you understand. That, what they believe to be their own individual and personal eccentricity, is very common and familiar and that lots of people are that way. As soon as the patient begins, gingerly, to tell me about the situations that bring on the anxiety, I add some brush strokes to his account, to show that I am aware of what they are talking about.

– When was the first time it happened? I ask.

– I was in a bus one day...

– You felt discomfort?

– Yes. I needed some air...

– Was it crowded and very hot?

– I was afraid I would faint...

– And you got off at the first stop.

– I couldn't stay in it. I got off as if someone was chasing me and got some air...

– And after that you never got on another bus.

– I try to avoid it ... I take taxis now. It's very expensive but I can't do anything else. In a bus I think I'm going to choke, that I'll faint...

– And be ridiculous.

– Exactly.

– Don't you feel discomfort in a taxi when you're in a traffic jam?

– Oh yes. I do. Once we stopped under a bridge, in a small tunnel and I wanted to open the door and run away. And the worst was when I saw I couldn't open the door, as we were too close to other cars...

2. The second step of treatment is to find the relation in the time of the first attack to some period of mental or physical distress. The first anxiety attacks generally occur during, or just after a period of stress. It could be a separation or divorce, a dismissal from work or a new job, a new position with greater responsibilities. It could be moving house or buying or building a new one. It is also frequently the illness or death of a person close to them. In particularly vulnerable people the first attacks can present themselves following minor events such as university exams or a rejection of a proposal of love.

Relating the attacks to distress, gives the patient the first feeling that they are not something only they are prone to, a weakness of theirs, but an illness that is due to a physical or mental distressed state. Sometimes the patient will deny it, saying that they have been through worse before without any problem having appeared, evidently to demonstrate how strong they are. They will often say:

— *Me, I'm strong. I've been through much worse. Everyone has said to me that I'm strong and that I'll never collapse. That everybody can get depressed except me ...*

— *You should know that strain and weariness accumulate. They add up over the years until when something that appears insignificant happens, the system falls apart. It's the last straw that causes it to disintegrate.*

It is something I often have to tell my patients. It is important that they should see the relation between the two. I must say in fact that they accept physical strain more easily than mental. This is why I emphasise the first. I don't really know why this is, except that in the domain of psychoanalysis, mental strain has been inculpated. In our society, mental stress has been connected to 'problems that cannot be solved', with unbalanced people. With people who need an analyst, a healer, a psychologist or whatever you want to call them. It counters the image of the independent individual who stands on his own feet.

3. The third step for dealing with the trouble is to accept that it is an illness. I prefer this to be in the presence of the accompanying persons, whether they are parents, a spouse or friends. I ask whoever comes with the patient to come into my office, and first of all ask them their opinion. What they think about the patient. Is there something wrong with the person or not. The most usual reply is:

—*Oh Doctor, there's nothing wrong. We've been to so many doctors, and for so many tests, really exhaustive but as you will have been told, nothing was found... It's all in the mind...*

At this point I become serious. As if I were going to have to announce some very unpleasant news.

— *That's exactly it. There is damage to the brain. It's an illness of the brain. There's nothing wrong with the heart, the stomach or the lungs but there is in the brain, which regulates and controls all the body's functions ...*

And I spell out the mechanism that causes anxiety attacks. It is astounding to see the expression on the face of the patient at that moment. Suddenly, they have been exonerated. They have been to doctors, hospitals, and left every time with the feeling that not only were their symptoms doubt but the panic was ignore that has been so distressing that it was paralysing. Until now, nobody has realised what they suffer. So far, the physicians had been condescending and told them not to worry! No–one had said, looking so serious and being so direct, that the person was truly suffering. No doctor had acknowledged the pain, both the mental and the physical. In the best case they nodded sagely and prescribed some sedative. In fact, most often they would take the companions aside, out of hearing of the patient, to say "… not to worry, it's nothing."

Now at last the patient is borne out to be right, in front of the relatives and escorts. In the most definitive manner, by a doctor, what they thought about their companion has been discredited. That person is not merely a complainer or worse, a sniveller. They are sick, with a serious disease that has ruined their life.

In fact, I go a step further, and say: "… this illness has crippled you." They are shattered at first, but I point out – still in front of the entourage – that the illness has caused social crippling. They can't circulate alone. They can't go wherever they wish. It means in essence that they have lost their liberty.

This strategy, acknowledgement of the illness in the presence moreover of the relatives, gains the psychiatrist the esteem of the patient. Although they have usually come to see him with many reservations, the doctor is now the great ally. And when this powerful alliance has been formed the next step may follow: medication.

4. Then **the fourth** step is to unfold the pharmaceutical strategy. It has to be explained in the patient's vocabulary, in terms they will comprehend. I often use examples from their work sector or that of the accompaniers. I describe the pathology of the illness and the ensuing goals of the treatment. For instance, to an auto mechanic I used an example I often make use of:

– *Because of the adversities of your life as well as your character, the battery we have in the brain was emptied. It was exhausted and could no longer control how easily the panic button of your organism may be pressed. It's an alarm system that is usually useless but nevertheless it makes us feel terribly agitated and anxious, together with cardiovascular symptoms and other systems that could be a minor problem for any of us.*

Therefore, the treatment has a twofold approach: first of all to replenish the battery and secondly to tighten the alarm button that has come loose, so that it cannot easily be pressed. The first is done with antidepressants and the second with anxiolytic drugs. This means the target of the antidepressants takes a long time to reach and requires constant administration to replenish the battery properly. If it is stopped too soon the battery may not be fully charged and so can easily empty again.

On the other hand, the anxiolytic, sedative drug will slow down the alarm button. So as to help the battery to be recharged, the alarm must not be activated too often. Therefore, a strong sedative dosage has to be administered. When the attack occurs the discomfort increases the anxiety, causing recycling which in turn leads to a peak of anxiety. This is why the dose of anxiolytic has to be substantial. It is the only way to avoid a triggering of the anxiety crisis and the panic attack.

Everyone, the patients and their company, understands that they have to be bold in the dosage of the sedative drugs as well as not to be in a hurry to stop the antidepressants. Those are the principal errors usually made in dealing with the illness of anxiety. The major problem lies in the widespread conviction that sedative drugs are bad for you and must consequently be taken as little as possible. On the other hand there is the belief that one must not depend on psychiatric drugs. One would think that they are administered to be enjoyed, like smoking or drinking or smoking pot.

It is time we advanced from the prejudices of the past, the days when every sort of psychiatric therapist defamed psychiatric drugs, being afraid they would be out of work. We must realise at last that just as medicine for the heart saves countless lives and improves the quality of life, what we call collectively psycho-drugs got 'mad' people out of asylums. Psycho-drugs also save people from suicide and have tens of millions smiling and happy, every day.

The key to treatment of anxiety attacks is precisely in the increased dosage of anxiolytic drugs and in lasting administration of antidepressants. The doses should be as strong as possible, without causing drowsiness or sleepiness. I explain to my patients from the outset that I do not want them to be drowsy but that also do not want them to have another attack. I explain that attacks can be prevented. The object is to have them feeling relaxed and not constantly with 'clenched teeth'.

Patients understand what I'm saying. It's usually only the relatives who object:

– *But, Doctor, isn't he/she going to be addicted to that medicine, and how to quit, later?*

I could say these are the standard questions heard. And my standard reply is:

– *At present that medication is absolutely essential. There will be no improvement without them. When our patient is better, in due course, they won't be indispensable so, we'll gradually lower the dose until they can be withdrawn. That is, if possible. I have to tell you from the outset that cases exist, where they are necessary for a very long time. However, the good news is that both the anxiolytic and the modern antidepressant drugs are perfectly safe. They are the safest sort of medication, with no side-effects. Millions of people all over the world take them, for years and years, without any noticeable side-effect. My advice to you is to relax and let your friend get on with their therapy so as to be relieved of the trouble torturing them.*

5. The fifth step is to restore our relation to a level of warmth. I give the patient my card with my mobile phone number and, insisting, in the presence of the accompaniers I strongly emphasise that the whole basis of the therapy rests on our communicating.

– *We'll work together to find the right dosage of the anxiolytic drugs. To begin with, you'll take what I think is the right one, but the wardrobe will be made to measure and you will be trying them on. Nobody can know the exact right dose needed. By staying in touch by phone, we'll be able together to find the proper one.*

– *When should I call you, Doctor?*

– *As soon as you start taking the medication. Ring me the next morning to tell me how you slept. You might not have had a good night or on the contrary not be able to wake up. We'll decide together how much anxiolytic medicine you have to have. The scenario is easier for the antidepressants. We start with minimal doses and increase them gradually, week by week.*

It's the 'togetherness' I underline. The doctor–patient cooperation model places the patient in the centre and the doctor as the collaborating partner who has complete understanding. The patient has at last found someone to be on his side, even against the relatives.

I must mention here that many of my colleagues do not like to give patients their mobile phone number, but I have learned from experience that when the physician is available for communication, patients rarely abuse of the facility they have been given. Furthermore, nowadays in the years these days of communications, if a patient feels shut away they can easily find where their doctor is hiding, however much he tries to.

What especially insecure patients do, usually, is to telephone once at the outset of the collaboration, just to make sure that the doctor is truly available. When that has been ascertained they calm down and not only no longer pester, they feel greatly improved security in general. Most of them enter my number on their mobile so as to feel that I am 'always there for them'. That too is part of the therapy. It must not be forgotten that most of them have been rejected by friends and family. The more the sufferers have asked for help, the more those close to them kept their distance and were not interested to help.

So that when somebody says: "I'm always there for you" they are grateful, and they relax. From the usual dismissive stance of the other specialists, summed up in the twin phrases: "there's nothing wrong with you, you needn't come back" to the opening of means of communication, there is a vast difference which the patient recognises and values accordingly.

Nevertheless, because the doctor–patient relationship has to be based on complete sincerity, from the start the doctor has to make things clear about the use of the 'phone:

– *There are times when the phone is switched off because I'm asleep or in a meeting or on an errand when I can't talk to anybody. In that case, call back later. Also, if I sometimes should sound abrupt, it's because I'm busy with something else, for instance on top of a ladder... I'm telling you now so you are not offended. I might ask you to ring me later. It doesn't mean however that I'm putting you off or that you're bothering me. In any case, even if I'm on holiday or travelling abroad it will always be possible to communicate.*

This last step, of offering constant communication, of addressing them familiarly and often using the word 'together' in talking to them, is in my opinion another aspect of the doctor–patient relationship. I often tell my medical students that Medicine is a difficult art. It does not only require memorising all the pharmacopeia, when they are applicable and their side–effects. One of the principal needs is to establish good relations with the patient and their entourage in order to gain their cooperation.

It is a fact that every day patients come to see me who have already visited other colleagues without success. Most have in fact obtained excellent prescriptions from these doctors. But their confidence had not been won. In consequence, either the patients had not even taken the medication at all or took a smaller dose because they were scared. Sometimes, while duly taking the medicine as prescribed, all the side–effects they had read about in the leaflet accompanying it. I once heard a patient say:

– Oh Doctor, as soon as I took the pill the previous doctor had given me, I was trembling like a leaf. I could not stay in bed and I couldn't sleep. And indeed I had read in the little paper that comes with the package where it said clearly that a side–effect of the medicine is tremor.

But tremor as side effect in this medicine is expected only as a light trembling of the hands, barely noticeable when the patient handles a cup of tea! Evidently the colleague she had seen had not explained the possible side–effects nor had told her what was in the instruction leaflet.

Some of the complaints I hear about colleagues are: 'He/she didn't pay any attention to me', 'didn't spend any time with me', 'didn't let me speak nor explain'. Or, 'wouldn't listen to me, the parent, who knows better'. The patients also sometimes say that the doctor wouldn't look them in the eyes. Or, that the doctor seemed too young or too old. That the doctor hadn't shaved, was dirty, wasn't wearing a clean white coat, the office was peculiar, and anything else imaginable that can affect the doctor–patient relation.

But, that is where the game is played for the treatment to succeed: To build a relationship among the doctor, the patient, and their companions. The doctor's obligation is in every instance to encourage them to express their worries and their objections to the recommended treatment. It is the surest way for the doctor to gain their confidence.

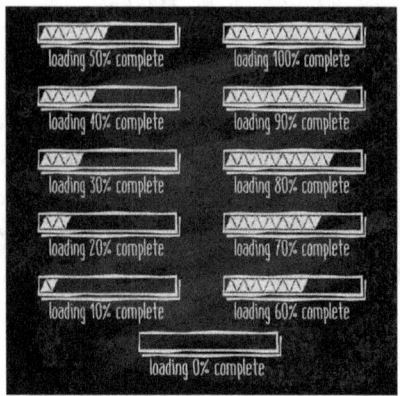

OBSESSIONS AND COMPULSIONS: DEFICIENCY OF PROGRAMME LOADING

WE OFTEN download new programmes on our computer or update other older ones. Usually, while this is being done the computer must stop what it was doing. This means we may for instance interrupt a letter we were writing, so as to download a new programme we have just heard is circulating. It is the same when we are notified that a programme we have in the computer needs updating or that we can check for viruses. We therefore stop what we were doing while waiting to download the new data.

We wait a while, downloading is completed, and we resume our normal work. This is an unavoidable annoyance in the course of the work we are doing yet. On the other hand, it helps to have better control of our computer and the advantages it may get from the Internet. We have secured it against viruses and it is ready to run the new programmes we want.

You will have noticed though that when the downloading of the update or the new programme is complete, the indication 'finish' or 'done' appears. We click on that and are then sure the job is done. Can you think what would happen if that indication does not appear? We would have to repeat the downloading process from the start.

The damage to the brain of obsessive–compulsive patients is apparently similar to this fault. The downloading of the programmes is not completed and there is no final indication of 'done' in the procedures of control and integration of fresh data. Since the patient is therefore not sure that the new data is stored in the 'hard disk' of their brain they are obliged to repeat the operation or the thought: they ask themselves "did I close the door properly? I'll take a look." They see it is shut but as soon as they leave, they doubt again. So they will check again, in order to update the data entered on the 'hard disk' of the brain. But they are still not sure, because they have not clicked on the 'finished' button and go back again and again. It is no use, however, since there is a problem with completing the procedure and the appearance of the closure indication, so they are never sure that the operation they just finished has truly been 'successful'.

Some patients make their own rules. They think "if I check seven times, then I will be sure", which is what they do and then stop worrying. However, in some cases at the moment obsessive–compulsives are checking, they have to interrupt this specific ritual because for instance the 'phone rang just then'. In such cases they have to start all over again. Another seven times!

I had a patient who, when washing his hands 13 times – that was the number he had chosen – had not to think of anything else. He had to concentrate on the hand washing. If, by bad luck, some unrelated thought passed through his mind, he had to begin the ritual again from the start. So it often happened that he spent hours washing his hands and using a bottle or two of liquid soap!

It is understandable that obsessive–compulsive patients are in consequence very little productive. Instead of occupying themselves with the real things they have to deal with, they occupy themselves with repetition of a thought or an action. Moreover, their thoughts and actions are in fact generally of secondary importance in the activity of a normal person. The act of 'locking the door' or 'switching off the boiler' is automatic in a normal daily routine, a simple process, something like checking the computer for viruses. But, in the patient's mind it takes on a principal role. All their attention is focused on that, in fact each patient has a particular chore. For some it is the boiler, for another whether the iron is still plugged in or the fridge door open.

Actually, the focusing starts out from a single action, a single idea. But as long as the patient is not treated, the problem tends to spread. It may set out from obsessive hand washing it may gradually extend to the same for taking a bath and then on to cleaning clothes. It may indeed reach the stage of throwing out their clothes after each use.

I cannot forget a patient, aged 25, who confided to me that he would throw out the washing machine every time he had used it. He collected a pile of clothes that he had worn outside the house only once and that he therefore considered as being 'dirty'. He washed them all loading the washing machine with successive batches, and when that was done, he threw it out. As I recall, he lived in a village in Epirus and threw the machines down a cliff near the village. (In those days, you see, there was no recycling.)

It is a typical case, because the poor guy was not well off, so as to cover his 'eccentricities'. He forced his parents to buy him new machines by otherwise being 'ill' and so beside himself that they were obliged to give in.

Also typical is that while obsessive–compulsive patients are basically aware that what they do is unnecessary and unreasonable, yet they cannot refrain from doing it. When it is an action, we call it 'compulsion' and an idea, an "obsession".

Compulsions, that is to say, are the repeated, excessive and illogical actions such as washing, locking, switching on/off, until the sufferer is sure. Obsessions are repetitions in the same way of superfluous and irrational ideas, such as 'I must make a wish for all to go well for me' or 'I mustn't go past a church in case I blaspheme' or 'I have to add up all the numbers on the plates of the cars that pass me', or even 'if an unpleasant thought crosses my mind, I instantly have to think of something pleasant', because otherwise things will go badly.

Both obsessives and compulsives usually execute a sort of ritual; something that is repeated, with no essence, just to be able to reassure the patient, just as we may make the sign of a cross when passing a church, mechanically, without the particular act having any meaning, relative to our degree of religious faith. In fact, some cross themselves every time they past a church, because otherwise they think that if they did not succeed, it will be bad for them.

I once saw a man on a scooter on the avenue, who was going much too fast, while, what's more, it was raining, let go of the handlebar to make the sign of the cross because he passed a church! I wondered at the time whether God would be pleased with that act or if He saw him from above, He would tell him in a thunderous voice "hands on the handlebar and your mind on the road not on churches…"

Patients realise these actions are needless and unimportant and their only objective is to lessen the anxiety the patient feels when he executes them. For example, some chew their fingernails when they are stressed. This brings them a moment's relief. If on the other hand, someone forbids them to bite their nails, it is certain their anxiety will reach a peak. They themselves know this perfectly well, which is why they do not even try to restrain themselves from performing the totally useless act.

The same goes for the other compulsions and obsessions. The patients know that if they try to avoid the irrelevant actions or the inconsequential and often childish thoughts, they will become so anxious that they will have no relief until they perform them. Hours might go by, without their being able to think of anything else.

One of my patients, when driving, would suddenly think: "Did I hit somebody at the crossroads I just passed without noticing?" Sometimes he would stop immediately and look all over the crossroads to make sure there was nobody injured or killed. Sometimes, if he was in a hurry, he did not stop and forced himself to go on, all the while knowing the doubt was unfounded. But he could not rid himself of it and once he had to go back after an hour's driving to reassure himself and put his mind at rest. Indeed, one day he had gone home in the evening and could not sleep because of this irrelevant and futile obsession. So he got up, flung some clothes on and went back to the crossroads that earlier he had not checked out scrupulously!

Such people are trapped inside themselves. They live in the restraints they themselves have imposed without wanting to, out of their insecurity. The core of obsession–compulsion lies precisely in personal insecurity. It is an insecurity usually cultivated by the parents. Parents, also without meaning to, pull the rug out from under the feet of their children or, more poetically, by clipping their wings. It is generally due to over–protectiveness, because they do not have a fundamental confidence in their children's abilities. In many cases among my patients there was a father, especially authoritarian, with high expectations from the child in particular, resulting in causing the child's insecurity. The latter usually led to the (protective) bonds of strict limits that obsession–compulsion imposes. Less frequently have I come across compulsive patients where the mother played the central role, and this was in cases of girls, but with exceptions of every rule. It must always be remembered that the investigation of the human psyche is full of surprises and reversals.

It is, of course, not enough for a father to be authoritarian and with high expectations to turn someone into a compulsive state. Most young people rebel against a parent of that sort. And, believe me, such rebellion is an absolutely healthy reaction. For a young person to become compulsive, not only must the parent's ambitions be acceptable, but also the acceptance in the course of time, of the impossibility or difficulty of reaching those goals. Usually, that is, the child who becomes compulsive initially identifies with the parent. They accept the plans made for them. At the same time they also accept the parent's doubt as to their capacity to succeed. In other words, they uncomplainingly accept the belittling from the parent, which implied lack of confidence on their part.

Uncomplainingly? Certainly not. The compulsions constitute the complaint. It is however, a protest without an open clash. Since the compulsion cripples the child, thus painfully punishing the ambitious parent. Of course, primarily it is the sufferer who is punished. This is the strategy of culmination of what we call 'passive aggressiveness'. In this case I aggress or attack the parent, passively, by not accomplishing what the parent expected from me.

Here it is worth pointing out the two fields in which obsessive–compulsive patient operates. It is both to punish the parent and at the same time is punishment for the sufferers themselves. Unfortunately, in the course of their life, the parents' place is taken by those who are close to them; spouse, in–laws, relatives, even the children, as well of course as the doctor, who is trying to help. Therefore, be careful not to press the patient, for if they interpret it as aggression, then the answer will be to increase the symptoms. Just as when exerting pressure on someone to quit smoking they may smoke more, in a compulsive patient it may exacerbate the compulsions. For the sufferer it is the only way they know to respond to aggression! Suffering, of course, more themselves. But they know that in this way, they are more trouble to their entourage.

A fifteen–year–old girl 'had a problem' with her strict father. Every time he criticised her, it fed her insecurity. In her troubled brain, this translated into insecurity about cleanliness. It transmuted into her feeling 'dirty' so, she had to go the bathroom right away to wash. She would dash off and wash herself for at least an hour. The other members of her family, including her father, could not use the bathroom all that time! Punishment of her father did not end there, as for every bath she took she used up some cubic metres of water, a whole bottle of shampoo and one of bubble–bath, as well as four towels that had to go to the wash immediately. The girl's skin was peeling off from frequent washing and she could not enjoy her life and the family, were in a living hell. They could not make any plans, because at any moment the girl might 'occupy' the bathroom for hours. They obviously could not invite anyone to their home, nor be in time for appointments. In both ways, the girl was a prisoner of her illness and, vice versa, so was her family.

This is where the secret lies in how to deal with obsession–compulsion. The patient must in no way be under pressure that will be interpreted as aggressiveness. They must be allowed, to take the initiative in their movements. All that can be done, is to show them how 'imprisoned' they are so, as to reinforce the motive to escape from their prison, which of course means, to make the keys available to them, to get out of the bars that surround them. However, on no account must those keys be given into their hands, nor any bars be unlocked for them, because then the illness will immediately forge new bars. It is the nature of the illness. In essence, the patient has to overcome the insecurities of their self. If we solve the problem for them it only confirms their insecurity.

Dealing with obsessive–compulsive patients takes a very long time and requires enormous tolerance and self–restraint. It is however, like any other difficult objective, a challenge that can give great satisfaction when eventually the sick person is released from the chains of torment of the illness.

What is as important in obsessive–compulsion disorder is that usually the pathological behaviour patterns spread, like ink stains. It starts out as a spot and in time takes over all the behaviour of the sufferer. As a tiny and insignificant 'spot' it may exist in a person for years, without causing any problem. How many people are there who have minor and limited fixations or compulsive 'eccentricities', that do not cause any problem in their everyday life, from the simple game of 'not stepping on the joints of paving stones' to taking their 'lucky pen' to important exams or interviews.

Actually, the various fetishes and lucky charms are a form of compulsion. They are customs, superstitions we call them, that we know basically have no powers. It is childish to knock on wood to avoid a misfortune we have just spoken about. Knocking on wood is evidently, not the way to prevent a cancer. Nor do the lucky charms that many coaches and athletes use, improve their performance or bring their team victory. However, the reason the habits are so prevalent, is that all those fellow humans of ours who turn to the 'metaphysical power' of those superfluous objects or acts, are basically afraid that if they do not perform those crazy and irrational commandments they will be exposed to disastrous scenarios. It is the insecurity inherent in them, initially instigating them. And then later, if not obeyed, they are afraid that something bad might happen. Besides, 'what's wrong with knocking wood'? If a person does it, their anxiety is soothed and they calm down right away, but if not, insecurity will gnaw at them until it is done. The resulting diminished anxiety reinforces the conviction that the act must always be performed, even if it is illogical.

Nonetheless, these 'normal' spots of obsession and compulsion may be activated under stressful circumstances and begin to spread. If, for instance, I lose my job or separate from my spouse, the game with the paving joints could become a nightmare! I would have to look at the ground all the time and then begin doubting whether I stepped on a joint by mistake. So, I have to go back and walk the same way again, taking more care. It can happen, and therefore walking outside the house would become torture, and for this reason the patient will not go outside at all.

The treatment

IT WAS INITIALLY observed that a tricyclic antidepressant drug, chlorimipramine may decrease compulsiveness. This is a break–through not only in the treatment but also in the theory of compulsion. Until then it had been believed that it was a bad habit, to be corrected only by education and pressure.

Thus, in the pre–drug era, treatments had been developed addressing behaviour solely, and they were therefore called 'behaviour treatments'. The key element of these treatments was exposure of the patient to the imagined danger. If for example they are afraid their hands may be dirty and wash them continually, the behaviour–therapist would make them put their hands in the dirtiest possible matter and then not wash them. Naturally, at the outset the patient with the 'dirty' hands is overcome by anxiety. The behaviour therapist however tries seduction, making light of the stress and phobias, for the patient to lessen the anxiety gradually. This is to give the patient the opportunity to acquire the certainty that, nothing disastrous is going to happen to them if their hands are 'dirty'.

These behaviour treatments, besides of being expensive – they required a personal therapist and multiple sessions – were ineffectual. They may have stopped the anguish of the 'clean hands', but the ingenious human brain finds other fields for the exercise of compulsive behaviour, such as locking/unlocking, or whatever our mind can imagine. Additionally, success in obsessions was very limited, because ideas are more difficult to be dealt with than actions.

In behaviour therapies the psychiatrists and psychologists of those days tried to persuade a patient not to repeat the act, not, that is to say, to download, again, a particular programme, even though they are not certain they have successfully completed it.

In many instances they managed to impel patients to work normally, whereas they still doubted whether they had downloaded some programmes: "I can do my work, even if I'm not sure my hands are clean."

What is achieved with medications is that every updating of the mind is complete, through to the appearance of the 'done/finished' button. The patient's mechanism sees that the procedure was completed and no longer feels it has to be repeated. Chlorimipramine thus acted on the whole spectrum of compulsions, diminishing the need to repeat actions. It was evident that it was a radical and aetiological treatment.

What was, however, strange was that whereas chlorimipramine is an effective antidepressant, the other antidepressants of the time did not have such good results. While treating depression, they had no effect on compulsions.

The particularity of chlorimipramine was that it is especially effective in serotonin activity. This leads to the conclusion that compulsion is connected to a serotonergic circuit in our brain.

This formation of serotonergic circuit must also be connected to the circuit, which is exhausted by depression as well. Because the reason is that it is fairly frequent for the phenomenon of compulsivity to present itself in periods of depression or general distress, to the extent that many believe that compulsive behaviour is a symptom of depression. It is a fact that depressive patients often, at some moment, present an obsessive or compulsive symptom.

On the other hand, compulsive symptoms may also be present in schizophrenia. It therefore seems that the serotonergic mechanism, which malfunctions in compulsivity, is independent from the one responsible for depression.

A further element supporting this theory is that the restoration of that independent mechanism requires a higher dosage and longer time of prescription of chlorimipramine or SSRIs (Selective Serotonin Reuptake Inhibitors) – newer antidepressants that selectively increase the action of serotonin. For example, while the usual dose of the first historically SSRI named fluoxetine, is 20 – 60 mg daily for the treatment of depression, to deal with obsessive compulsive disorder, a much higher dose may be required.

I had an extremely compulsive patient. His life was a hell because the thoughts that came to his mind were not only of the prohibited kind, they were disastrous. He had a stall in an open air market and if someone looked him in the eye, the thought would come to him was to use the knife he had in his hand and slit that person's throat. The picture was so vivid that he was afraid it could really happen, but, however much his logic told him that he would never execute such mad acts, he could not stop the thoughts from pestering him constantly. It was not only a pest — they did not only make him unhappy — they also prevented him from thinking clearly and concentrating on his work.

After years of suffering, at some point he decided, or rather he found the courage, to seek assistance from a specialist. He described his condition, without daring to describe his thoughts. The description of the symptoms was however characteristic: an irrational thought that invades the mind, obstructing the normal thought process, in essence not allowing him to pay attention or concentrate. It is a thought the patient is aware of, knows it is illogical but that he cannot get rid of and is thus very troublesome. This is the definition of obsession.

I therefore prescribed fluoxetine, in a gradually increasing dosage. The patient began to feel relief from the daily torture of his thoughts. Indeed, he felt so much better when the treatment's dosage was increased, that of his own initiative he reached the point of taking 200 mg fluoxetine a day! He has been taking this large dose for many years and it improved his efficiency to such an extent, that he himself will not even consider reducing it. It is noteworthy on the other hand that this high dosage did not bring him to a manic state. As he himself assesses his symptoms, it brings 95% relief and he is deeply grateful to me, but that is not yet complete. There remains a 5% which I urge him to deal with, with his own powers of his mind.

It is a fact that, with the help of the medication, many patients' symptoms are lessened and they are able to fight their crazy thoughts and the insecurity that drives them to repeat superfluous acts. Pharmaceutical treatment opens the way to a better and easier confrontation of this troublesome illness. Additionally, as the symptoms subside thanks to the medicine, the sufferers begin to be convinced they do have a biological illness and that it is not their fault as most of them believe, as well as their entourage.

Compulsion is not an eccentricity of their character, nor a bad habit they must overcome. It is not something they can control. Obsession and compulsion is something they cannot overmaster because, quite simply, it is the product of a fault in a circuit of their brain. It is a circuit improved by medicines that reinforce serotonergic transmission.

I tell them that the medicine helps to complete, ('done' or 'finished'), the downloading of various everyday programmes, so that from there on the patients can fight their insecurities, which is to say the uncertainty whether the downloading has been correctly effected.

As I said earlier, schizophrenic patients also sometimes present symptoms of compulsion, in fact in the initial stages of development of the illness. This was the reason for the view to be expressed that the symptomatology of compulsion, was a manner of a person's defence against the emergence of schizophrenic symptomatology. It is however obvious that there is a relation between the mechanism that causes compulsive symptomatology with the mechanism that produces delusions, the characteristic symptom of schizophrenia. That is to say that it appears that in some patients the serotonergic mechanism of compulsion is exhausted by similar dopaminergic stimulations. The excess of dopaminergic stimulation causing delusions – whose mechanism was expounded in the chapter on schizophrenia – is damages connected to serotonergic circuits. These are the circuits responsible for compulsiveness. This is how some patients who are sensitive to these serotonergic neuron circuits, present compulsions.

The logic of connected mechanisms says that, if schizophrenia is treated with antipsychotic drugs, it is to be expected that the compulsive symptoms will be controlled. It does happen in most of the cases. This is why psychiatrists who see things from a psychoanalytical point of view say that compulsions constitute a mental defence in the schizophrenic process. When the schizophrenia is pharmaceutically controlled, the defence is superfluous and consequently diminishes.

However, as things are not always simple in medicine, some drugs that treat schizophrenia at the same time have a negative effect on the serotonergic mechanisms controlling compulsive symptomatology. Thus, while treating schizophrenia with those particular drugs, compulsions may be triggered in these schizophrenics.

On the other hand, to show how difficult the practice of medicine is, we know that the drugs reinforcing the serotonergic mechanisms of compulsions exacerbate schizophrenia. That is, when chlorimipramine and the more recent antidepressants are administered to schizophrenics, they provoke exacerbation of schizophrenic symptoms. It is another indication that the two mechanisms, of schizophrenia and compulsions, are connected operationally but are independent.

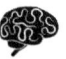

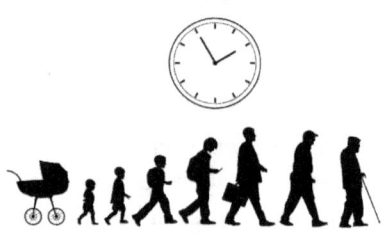

DEMENTIA: AN UNAVOIDABLE DETERIORATION?

AS IS ALL in this futile world, the brain has a limited resistance to the passage of time. Of course, in animals nature is able to surpass the time limits of resistance of the particular materials they are made of, with the method of replacing them with new ones of the same structure. Cells are constituted of construction material that, in the course of time, break up and are replaced. In this way the cell remains functional, despite the wear and tear of the proteins and other structural elements constituting it.

Theoretically, the break up and re–assembly of the materials may go on endlessly. In practice however, the system is not perfect. Of course demolition and rebuilding does not only sustain structures; they also help the organism to adapt to new circumstances. On the other hand though, errors occur all the time in this complicated process. Some protein or other will not be perfectly demolished and will remain within the cell like useless rubbish, resulting in the cell gradually filling with trash and becoming ineffective and being deadened.

We think this is the mechanism by which some brain cells are destroyed in Alzheimer's disease. It appears in fact that some people genetically, do not have the suitable enzyme for breaking up a protein into small pieces for them to be eliminated as waste from the cells. Thus, cells gradually fill with large fragments of that protein that cannot be eliminated. Finally of course these cells die, filled with the deficient metabolised ruins of this specific protein.

Another, perhaps more frequent, cause of death of brain cells is an inadequate blood supply. The heart may at times briefly interrupt its function, which we feel as arrhythmia. Tiny clots then form in the heart which, when transferred to the brain, block small vessels in the brain, causing small and very often unnoticed vascular episodes. In this case we are talking about multi–infarct dementia.

This is how in brain imaging of many aged patients small dead areas are observable. The damage may not be at spots causing motion problems and hence are not revealed in a clinical neurological examination. These deficiencies however, when they add up, bring about difficulties in fine motional functions, at the same time hindering mental functions. They give the patient the aspect of senility, that is to say showing a disturbance of memory, as well as judgment.

A practical and sensitive test that reveals problems in the coordination of mental operations such as senile patients, often present is the sketching of a clock. Draw a circle on a piece of paper and ask the person suspected of being senile to put in the numbers representing the hours around the perimeter of the circle, exactly as on a clock face. It seems easy enough but you may be astonished that most old people find it very difficult and usually make mistakes.

The next step is to ask them to draw the hands of the supposed clock to show 'ten past ten' for instance. This exercise is not quite so easy, for it requires ability of perception as well in abstract thought. It is a simple test for the existence of problems in brain function related to senility. Indeed, it reveals troubles even in patients who do not have other visible elements of deficient intellectual function.

With this simple test I have often discovered and documented mental disturbances in old people, who initially seemed to be perfectly well. What happens in the initial stages is that some clever aged persons learn how to cover up their deficiencies. The most usual way is to give answers approximately:

– *How many children do you have?*

– *As many as God gave me.*

– *Where do you live?*

– *Where I've been living all this time. Where my children were born and brought up. It's not a big house, Doctor, but it's enough for us.*

When hearing such vague replies, one should suspect senility. The simple test of the clock would show and confirm the diagnosis.

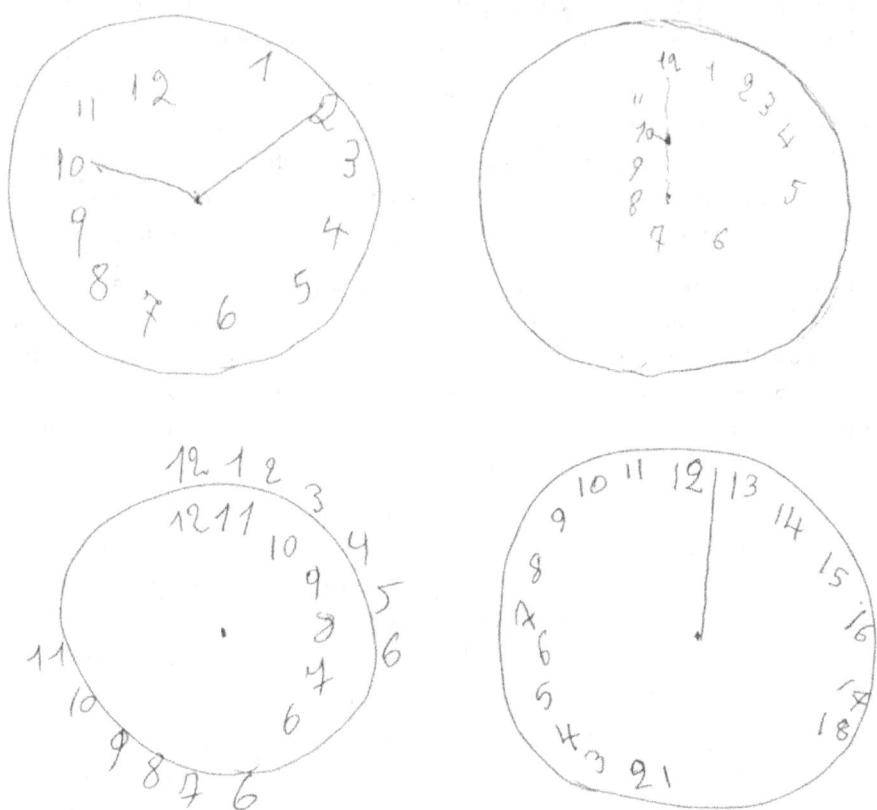

I cannot forget a retired lawyer who was brought to me by his daughter because she had noticed some odd behaviour. Her father lived alone, looked after by a daily maid. He went around quite independently and saw to all errands himself. Recently however he had not been buying the items on the list the maid had given him for the shops, but different things. Whenever she asked him why, he always found an excuse:

– *Mr. Jordan, why did you buy apples? I wrote oranges on the list.*

– *The apples were fresher.*

– *Yes, but I need the oranges to make your morning juice.*

Then, when Mr. Jordan tried to draw the clock as I asked him, he was in great difficulty. At first he giggled, saying it was too childish, but then he couldn't get going. When he concentrated he began writing all the numbers from 1 to 12 in the same semicircle of the supposed clock. When he was done, he realised there was something wrong but he still couldn't see his mistake.

I want to say here that this simple test is much more useful than MRIs that are so popular. These costly imaging methods give a picture of the anatomy of the brain. But they say nothing about its functioning. I myself have seen extensive atrophies in brain imaging, without however having been corresponding significant deficiencies in their functionality.

The symptoms

MOST BRAIN cells are responsible both for the storing of data and for their processing. In consequence, when they die they lead a person to loss of memory, indeed of the recent time. This means that they cannot remember what they just did. The patient cannot remember where they put their keys or their money. In fact what often happens is that when they look for them and don't find them, they think somebody took them.

Old people often thing that someone comes into their home and steals from them. It results in their making up a whole story in their imagination – which they do not lack – that at night someone creeps unseen into the house and robs it. At times indeed, they may target some particular relative or neighbour as being the burglar.

There was a case where it was difficult for me not to laugh when a senile old lady confided to me that a female neighbour of hers was stealing her clothes, shoes, even underwear. "That dirty woman wears them and then days later she brings them back, filthy…" Evidently the patient hid her dirty clothes in various parts of the house, instead of putting them in the clothes' basket and found them days later, accusing her neighbour.

Delirium and delusions makes senile people more suspicious and paranoid so that they hide keys, money and anything of value in the most unbelievable places in their home. Their children come to me to say they can't find their father's or mother's hiding places of their health or savings deposit booklets. As, nowadays, many elderly people have someone from outside the family looking after them, this paranoid tendency makes it more difficult for their relatives.

I have, of course, also had experience of such caregivers taking advantage of and exploiting the situation. Certain such people looking after senile patients have found ways to embezzle sums of money, or even to convey monies to third parties, or also to become included in the will and the inheritance of the elderly person.

I remember an old lady, the widow of a big businessman. She had no children or immediate family. She had a foreign live-in maid. Every month the family solicitor who managed the assets, would bring the old lady a substantial sum and give it to her. So as to get her hands on the money, the maid would suggest a game of cards. Naturally the senile patient always lost and the maid in this way had made a lot of money, the amount of which the old lady could not evaluate. One day, a distant niece of the patient appeared on the scene and the maid went back to her country. It was finally discovered that the woman had in this way extracted more than two million euro!

In another instance, the maid persuaded the elderly lady to give an apartment to the maid's son, whose the lady was godmother. The transfer was made in secrecy. No one in the family knew anything about it. It was discovered, after the old lady's death, when it was found that the flat had been given away.

To avoid such things happening, I always recommend to the family, as soon as dementia has been found, to address a court of justice so that the patient's legal competence should be restricted. This makes everything clear and indisputable by all.

It unfortunately happens frequently, that after the death of some elderly person the heirs quarrel amongst themselves, claiming that some of them had exploited the incompetence of the senile relative.

What almost always happens is that the relatives who take over the care of old people also manage their income. This can be with a simple power of attorney or, worse, not even that. In some small towns or town quarters the bank itself will hand over the elderly person's pension to a child or relative who looks after them, without any formal power of attorney. This means that the situation continues in a murky legal framework.

However, when I tell the relatives to proceed to obtain judicial assistance in the legal status of their aged relative, they say they haven't got the heart to do that. Most of them unfortunately think of it as a hostile act against the relative for the court of law to declare that person incompetent, that it is humiliating.

The truth is, however, just the opposite. The court's decision protects the old person, their assets and their rights. Senile patients are extremely vulnerable. They feel helpless, alone and unprotected, resulting in their being easy victims of exploitation. Whoever undertakes their care should resort to judicial assistance before it is too late for both the patient and the caregiver. The latter is indeed most important, because often relatives and friends who look after an old person and manage their assets have got into a lot of trouble without deserving it. The general belief is that, if the job is done correctly and with the best intentions, it suffices to protect us from legal complications.

However, I have seen instances, though, of relatives appearing after the death of the elderly patient, who had never done anything for them while the patient was alive, and who not only disputed the will, but also accused the person looking after them of criminal neglect, acts and omissions, even that this led to the person's death. If the caregivers had resorted in time to judicial assistance, nobody could accuse them that for example the patient had not been taken to such-and-such a famous medical centre for hospitalisation, or, on the contrary, for the reasons for the operation that cost the patient their life.

The simplest thing I have seen, that makes me recommend immediate resort to a judicial declaration of legal incompetence is the case of a daughter and sole heir of a little old lady whom I had examined in hospital before she died. I visited her in the framework of the psychiatric service I was offering at the time to the General Hospital. The old lady was anxious and confused, and after ascertaining that she suffered from an organic brain disorder, evidently in the domain of dementia, I prescribed therapy. When her mother died, the daughter told me that she discovered to her surprise that her mother's sole asset, the small house she lived in, in a poor quarter, had been 'donated' a year ago to the maid, a foreigner. It was clear to me – from my experience that already since a year before, the mother had not had proper judgment. That was why she had given away the house to the woman who was looking after her then. The house that she had acquired with her husband, through hard work and sacrifices and was destined for the daughter, her only child, who had been there before, looking after her every day. How could the daughter now claim that her mother was of disturbed mind, since at the same time her daughter had been taking the money of her mother's pension based on a power of attorney the mother had issued when she was supposed to be of sound mind?

The area of dementia is very murky and therefore needs to be clearly delimited before it is too late. On the other hand, a doctor's estimate as to past circumstances is most difficult and can be confuted. Besides, it is typical of dementia that there are periods of lucidity in the mental operations of the patient. Thus, at the outset at least, there are usually periods when the patient has clear judgment. Consequently the doctor cannot testify to the precise moment of commencement of incompetence for legal self-responsibility.

I shall mention here two personal instances of mine, to show what a difficult position a doctor can find himself in:

When I was starting my practice a man brought his father to see me, who presented signs of acute senility. In good faith I prescribed a drug that at the time was indicated for dementia. I wrote on the prescription, as I was obliged to do, that the diagnosis was 'dementia'.

A year later I was summoned for interrogation. One morning I did not go to work and went to the office of the examining judge, where I was told that there was an accusation against me! The old man's relatives – he had since died – were quarrelling over the validity of the will. The son had given as evidence my diagnosis on the prescription for the drug, with the premise that when the father had made the will he had been senile. The lawyer for the other side was suing me for 'issuing a false medical attestation'. Therefore, if I was unable to prove that my now deceased patient had been senile when I prescribed the medication, his son's claims would be nullified.

It is obvious I was all of a sudden in a very tight spot: dealing with lawyers, law courts, endless hours wasted, but above all I had to defend myself, with proof that was extremely difficult to do.

In the second case, I was asked to visit an elderly woman in a nursing home, to say whether she was senile. I found an 80–year old, bedridden. She could barely communicate and her mental capacity was evidently in a state of complete dissolution.

It would be natural to conclude that she was suffering from dementia. As however I am suspicious in such instances, I try to examine every aspect. So I asked to see what medication the lady was being given and found that she had been given antipsychotic drug which had evidently provoked severe physical as well as mental suppression. A colleague had had this drug administered when she was first admitted to the home and, as was natural, she was anxious it had been given to tranquilize her. But, they had continued to administer it without thinking whether it was indicated. I told them to stop the drug and saw the old lady again a month later.

Her condition surprised not only me but also the relative of hers who came with me. She was a different person! She had got up, was walking, with some assistance and, mainly, she was communicating again. She had traces of senility but, in no way could she be designated legally incompetent.

The treatment

IT IS TO BE expected that for each illness the chapter of treatment is eminently up to date. What is said to be incurable today may soon be treatable. At the time of writing this book, in that sense dementia, from whatever cause whether Alzheimer's or vascular is practically classed among the incurable illnesses.

In cases of loss of brain cells due to vascular malfunction, what can be done is to forestall damage by preventive measures. Timely care should be taken for the health of the arteries, reducing cholesterol and blood pressure, as well as for good functioning of the heart. The timely implant of a pacemaker and anti–coagulants can forestall many instances of multi–infarct, vascular dementia.

For Alzheimer's, on the other hand, the timely modification of the metabolism of a certain apoprotein is necessary. To date no such therapy has been found. A vaccine that a few years ago had shown encouraging results proved to have bad side effects. If effective therapy is found, one's genes will have to be examined in good time so as to know which people need it. The way to find out who has a genetic predisposition to the illness is known today but I do not consider it of use to track down possible candidates. Why should somebody know that they might be senile in their old age? Since nothing can be done to avert the process there is no reason to live under this chronic threat. The poor candidates could die from some other cause before then, happy, without the dread of eventual senility.

The medication existing today may temporarily help one's memory, but they are not at all effective against the deterioration of the brain cells that brings about dementia. They moreover have side effects for quite a lot of old people. Let it also not be forgotten that they are very expensive drugs and that once treatment is begun, they have to be taken all the time until death, for if they are interrupted the little improvement in memory will disappear right away.

Another pre–emptive of dementia, which is talked about a lot, is mental exercise. What people are most afraid of, now that it is most possible that their life expectancy will exceed 65 years, is that they will lose their mental agility. Most of them therefore, try to keep their brain in 'good shape'. They solve crossword puzzles, play cards, exercise with memory quizzes and anything else that is thought to keep the brain from becoming 'rusty'.

It is of course very difficult to make a scientific evaluation, whether any mental exercise can forestall the natural deterioration of the brain. What is certain is that mild physical exercise, by being good for the arteries and the heart, also helps the brain to function.

However, as in the case of physical exercise, where it has been shown that intensive strain may harm the articulations and the cardiovascular system, in mental exercise to excess may be deleterious. In theory at least, it is possible that in persons with a genetic defect in the breaking up of the apoprotein produced by those cells, their constant use may bring on their degradation sooner. In other words, their usage may 'burn up' the brain cells, in persons constantly occupied with mental exercises. Such a scenario is fairly plausible since it is known that in general brain cells are not renewed. I say jokingly to those I know who are worried lest they end up senile: "Don't worry. If you should suffer from dementia it won't be a problem for you personally. It will be a problem for those who will have to look after you at that time. You yourself will be perfectly happy."

It must, on the other hand, be borne in mind that patients appearing to be suffering from dementia but are not happy, may very well be suffering from depression. It could be in the early stages of dementia, when parallel depression makes the senility seem more severe, or it may be depression alone, that gives the impression of dementia. The latter instance is called 'pseudo–dementia'.

Usually, when a patient with real dementia is asked a question, he/she tries to answer. The answer may be wrong, it may be a generality, or a whole fabrication may be invented in the effort to satisfy the interlocutor.

To the question how many children they have and what their names are I have heard a variety of replies:

Some haphazard number, with a little laugh of embarrassment.

– *Lots, or enough children.*

– *As many as God gave me.*

– *In those days we had a lot of children because they helped in the work.*

The patient with dementia seeks the right answer. They look around to find a clue, they ask their accompaniers to help.

The depressive on the contrary, does not care if it's the right answer. They are imprisoned in the world of despair and can see nothing outside it. Very often they don't answer, or if pressed will say something like: "leave me alone", "I'm not interested in examination". However, things are not always so clear. A differential diagnosis between dementia and pseudo–dementia is not always easy.

One day a colleague sent me a 65–year–old lady to be hospitalised, telling me that she had been depressive in the past, but that she now gave the impression of dementia. The patient arrived at the hospital in an ambulance. She could not walk and had no contact with the environment. Her husband told me that she was in this state since she sold her business, which she had managed for 25 years. She was a very active person but who, in the past year had ceased any professional activity.

– *We have no children, so we have no obligations. At first my wife asked me to travel. We took some journeys for a while, but it tired me because, Doctor, I'm older than her and I have a heart and kidney problem. I don't want to be too far from my doctors. Also, I've been retired for years and I'm used to staying at home, for all the time my wife was a businesswoman.*

– *So you shut her up at home.*

– *Well, yes, but then she stopped being interested in anything, she didn't talk, nor could she do anything about housework. First she forgot to do the shopping, then she couldn't do the cooking and now she can't even look after herself. Now she just lies in bed and can't even walk. She doesn't understand what is said to her and, of course, she wears diapers, because she doesn't even know when she has to go to the toilet.*

When I saw her, she did indeed appear to be in the last stages of dementia. She had no contact with the environment. To whatever was said to her she responded with a blank look. It was as if she did not see you. My first reaction was 'what are we going to do with this patient in the University Clinic?' There's nothing we can do for her. She needs only nursing care, which she would have in a nursing home. My only reason for keeping her, to try to help with drug treatment, was her past history of depression, which my colleague had given me. I thought that although she was suffering from dementia, she could also be suffering from a degree of depression that aggravated the clinical picture of her dementia.

So I started giving her antidepressants. Treatment was not having results and I began doubting whether I was doing the right thing. On the other hand, there was anyway nothing else I could do for her. But the nursing staff were protesting, because they were not used to caring for bed–ridden patients. Not knowing what else to do, I increased the dosage of antidepressants excessively.

To everyone's astonishment, the patient began recovering. As if she was born again. She looked alert, she started talking and getting up and about. I need not say that when she left the clinic, two months later, she was a different person. It had nothing to do with dementia. It was as if the patient had returned from hell. The lady and her husband were so grateful that for three years she came to the Department every Monday morning with pastries for the patients and the staff! She herself was so well that she began occupying herself with her town's public affairs, in fact successfully.

Ever since, I have been treating many patients who were in the early stages of dementia with antidepressants. In some I see improvement in their cognitive function. I therefore believe that since we do not yet dispose of an effective therapy or preventive treatment for dementia, it is worthwhile to try an antidepressant therapy, at least for patients whose symptoms resemble depression such as what we typify as psychomotor retardation, being more emotional, apathetic or disinterested.

Whatever its type of dementia, we are going to have to deal with ever more cases in the years to come. As the population overcomes simple health problems, it will reach to a greater age and all the more of our fellow human beings will come to the point of deterioration of their brain that presents symptoms of dementia. It is to be hoped that an effective way of at least preventing Alzheimer's disease will be discovered. Of course, in regard to the more general deterioration of the vessels and disturbance of blood circulation, which is unavoidable in advanced age, the legend of Dorian Gray and eternal youth will continue to be a dream, out of the reach of all mankind.

Every time I am going to be sad because I feel I'm growing old, I think that if there were no decay, nor death, there would be no need for new birth. The show must go on. Unfortunately for our vanity, it will go on even better after us. As the world goes round, the evolution that gave birth to us, when we are dead will give birth to something better.

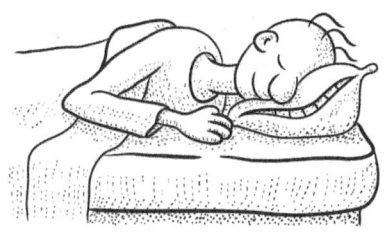

SLEEP: AN OBLIGATORY 'RESTART'

COMPUTERS ALWAYS annoy me, first because they have no judgment and so cannot understand what I want to do. The second annoyance is that every so, often when I have updated a programme or downloaded a new one, while I am impatient to run it, they ask me to do a 'restart'. When I complained to a friend of mine, an expert in computers, about this bothersome demand of the machines, she made this comparison: when you put a new element in a structure, even if it's just a brick, if your mind resembled today's computers you would have to close your eyes and then open them again so as to register the new completed picture of the structure in your memory. That is to say, for the new elements to be built in there has to be new completed loading of the whole. Or, to use the language of computer users, to add something to my 'boot' I have to take it off and put it back on again, that is 'reboot'.

It seems however that unfortunately the same applies to our brain, and not only ours but all animals who have a brain, from cockroaches to humans. For all brains to be able to continue functioning, for more than 20 hours, and to be able to process new data, have to close down and restart. Otherwise the brain does not have the capacity to receive nor of course to process new data.

It is a fact that sleep is more indispensable than food. No animal can go without sleep for more than few days at a time. Humans, for instance, whereas they can do without food for a number of days, cannot stay awake for more than seven to nine days. When it reaches its limit, it will produce hallucinations, mental confusion and finally will suddenly fall asleep irreversibly, as if the 'switches' of the brain had abruptly 'switched off'.

We have all experienced this sudden 'switching off' of our brain. When, we try to stay awake but our eyes – our brain in fact – close. If for instance we are having a good time until late at night and want to stay awake, without our meaning to, our eyelids close. Or the worst of all, and of course extremely dangerous, is to realise we are falling asleep while driving, although we are trying to avoid it in every way. It has in fact been calculated that 13% of accidents happen due to insufficient sleep.

The importance for the brain to shut down after some time of operation is shown in dolphins, the two hemispheres of whose brain shut down successively, the one after the other. This is because dolphins cannot let go and sleep because they have to come out of the water every so often to breathe. In this way, while one hemisphere sleeps, the other, that is awake, undertakes to lead the animal periodically to the surface. After a time the procedure is reversed, so that the other hemisphere could sleep. Thus, it seems that nature has been able to manage everything in its evolution except for one thing: to keep the brain of animals in constant operation without sleep.

What sleep does, therefore, is not to give the animal rest, as was once thought. What it needs to do is evidently to perform certain indispensable operations. Sleep is not a period of rest for muscles, it is a period when the animal's brain incorporates its experiences and the data of the immediately preceding stretch of time into its programmes.

It is evident that during sleep the brain performs indispensable jobs for its continuing normal functioning, such as filing and evaluating the new data. To accomplish this function the brain has to disconnect temporarily from the environment, just as the computer has to shut down and reboot.

But for every animal to accomplish the disconnection from the external surroundings, it has to find a safe and comfortable space. Find a place where its brain can be isolated, with no danger of being eaten by some enemy, nor freezing, nor being burned by the sun, nor drowning.

There is no doubt that sleep makes human beings more vulnerable to their enemies. Additionally, when asleep, muscle tone is diminished as well as diverse natural functions slowed down.

Moreover, muscle tone is relaxed so that the brain can perform its internal procedures that are needed, without this being apparent. For instance, to file planned movements without their being muscularly expressed. Something like jobs being done by the computer without showing on screen. In fact, during a period of sleep, the brain functions are particularly intensive. If during that time the muscles were not paralysed there would be intense disorderly and possibly violent body movements.

The architecture of sleep

SCIENTIFIC STUDY of sleep began with the recording done by the electroencephalogram (EEG) which concurrently records muscle tone and eye movements. The polygraph record of those three elements is called a hypnography or polysomnography.

Study of the hypnogram has shown that sleep includes two totally separate states. These states alternate in a specific manner, making what we call the architectural diagram of sleep. The usual scenario for an adult is for the activity of its cortex to diminish gradually from the moment they fall asleep. The EEG is co-ordinated and slow waves are recorded.

This stage of slow waves as they are called is suddenly interrupted by a 'paradox' stage of sleep, of Rapid Eye Movements or REM. At this stage the EEG records an intense brain activity, while at the same time muscle tone is almost nil. The only exception is the eye movement muscles that move the eyes rapidly in different directions. Breathing also becomes irregular and intense autonomic activity is noticeable: tachycardia, sweating and erection.

Dreams

IF SOMEONE is woken at the REM stage it is very probable that he or she will say they were having a dream. It appears that during this stage of sleep the experiences of the preceding period of alertness are classified. That is to say that all that was experienced during the day is seemingly stored in a temporary memory. This is too full at some point to be able to process more new information. In comparison, one may imagine that the data collected by our computer are temporarily stored in the 'desktop'. At some point the desktop fills up and can no longer store and process any more data. Data collected have to go to the archive, to the various files in our long-term memory, to leave empty space in the desktop for new data.

So, when the desktop is full, the brain gets sleepy and goes to sleep. And then it seems that during the REM phase of sleep, the files in the 'store' of long-term memory open, to receive the information collected during the day.

During the time this active procedure of storage and classification lasts, memories emerge from the past, combine with the recent and are re–classified. If the person is wakened at this time, they may remember pieces of experiences and images of the recent, as well as of the past time. The pieces usually relate to the experiences of the foregoing day. In this way something that was on our mind the previous day may in the REM phase we may re–process related past experiences, fears and anxieties they provoked, as well as proposals for their solution that we have in our memory.

Something, therefore, does not come into our sleep uninvited. I had evidently been thinking of it the day before and so in the night, while asleep, it had to be classified. That is why I dreamed of it. It is for this reason alone; that dreams have a value. They 'betray' the thoughts of the previous day, they betray our anxieties and aspirations, even those we do not want to admit to ourselves. Even those, that is to say, we wish to bury because they are impermissible and upset us.

Unconnected images come to our dreams which, however, generally have some connection to what was experienced or thought about the day before. Many people try to draw information about the future from these unconnected images. It is to be expected, since the images appearing in our dreams relate to whatever we have on our mind.

It is, however, obvious that dreams cannot have any prophetic capacity. It is simply that in this deficient, accidental and unconnected display of images we project, what we would like to hear about our future.

This is how the myth has arisen that dreams are prophetic. Unfortunately though, they have no more significance than clouds and their formations or the dregs of a Greek coffee and the flight of birds, from which for centuries the ancient augurs read the omens.

At the slow waves stage it appears that some coordination of the brain takes place. It is in fact noticeable; that, at the beginning of sleep, the slow waves are longer and more intense, whereas while sleep proceeds, in the subsequent cycles they become more superficial. This is a little like ploughing or combing one's hair. At the beginning of sleep the deep ploughing is done or the general arranging of the hair, while in the following cycles the details are attended to.

The operation of classifying and arranging of fresh experiences during sleep also explains; why young organisms need more sleep, because they have a greater volume of new data. A baby and later an infant are inundated with new experiences. Everything is new to them and they have to create categories and files in which to store what they experience for the first time. An older person has fewer new experiences and representations and the files have long been familiar.

It is not in fact a simple classification. It is also a re-evaluation of the allocation of data and representations to the files already opened. Furthermore, during sleep the connection among representations is also made. These shortcuts are consolidated and re-evaluated during sleep. For the programmes we worked out during the day, with our new experiences to be incorporated in our brain and become part of its 'arsenal' for whenever they will be needed, the brain has to have sleep. It has to shut down and reboot, fitting the new programmes into the rest already existing and 'running'.

Every time we sleep, the programmes are re-evaluated, according to the fresh experiences of the day before. Sometimes their filing can even change. Sleep is consequently of the greatest importance for the functioning of the brain. It is not merely a period of rest for the body and the mind.

Insomnia

BESIDES AGE, how long we sleep also has to do with each individual's idiosyncrasy. Some people need many hours of sleep, while others 'manage' with less than 6 hours in 24. In fact, this sentence holds the key to curing insomnia. Sleep is a necessity for the organism. If the organism is satisfied with fewer hours of sleep, there is no reason to press the person to sleep longer. I tell my patients who complain of insomnia, that I wish I could sleep less. I would actually have more hours for living.

There is however, unfortunately, the attitude that plenty of sleep is necessary and is therefore what every person should have. Many people worry every day whether they will be able to sleep as long as they 'think they should'. This thought alone, will affect the proper pattern of their sleep. They do not sleep deeply, because the anxiety brings interruptions and makes going back to sleep more difficult. So it affects the architecture of sleep and in the morning that person does not feel they slept well and their sleep is not refreshing. They will usually complain that they could not have a relaxed sleep and as night time approaches begin worrying that again they will not be able to sleep.

— *At night fall I think my time of martyrdom is approaching… a fifty-year-old told me.*

— *My bed has become an instrument of torture. I dread it like the devil does incense. I've tried everything, exercise, a warm bath, hot milk, herbal tea and herbs, relaxation… Nothing does any good. When I go to bed I can think one thing only: "Today again you won't be able to sleep." The clock next to me sounds like a hammer in my ears. I look at the time every so often… and think how many hours I have left before seven, when I have to get up. It's a real torture... and as you can imagine... I'm in a terrible state in the morning. It lasts all day. Doctor, give me a good night's sleep and I'll put up a statue of you."*

When I asked him if he had tried taking a sleeping pill, he said he had done that too.

– I took half one day, that a doctor friend of mine recommended to me, but it didn't do any good. My insomnia is not cured by medicines.

– No, it probably won't but nor will it help at all, with half of what your friend suggested. The level of your anxiety, of how wound up you are, when you go to bed is so high, that most certainly a higher dose is necessary for you to relax and sleep.

– But if I take a higher dose will I be able to wake up in the morning?

– Leave that to me, dear friend. There are medicines today that have completely left the organism in a few hours. Pilots take them, to sleep as long as they have to and then fly their plane perfectly.

The next question is usually whether the medication is habit–forming, and if they will depend on them. Will they have to take them for the rest of their life? And are they bad for the memory, as they read somewhere... Some also have the example of their grandmother who 'takes a sedative every night of her life and whenever it was tried to wean her she couldn't sleep.'

–Yes, but one didn't become two or three, as you are afraid it might. And if you'd like to know, she could have stopped, if she had done it very gradually. What's more, as you will have seen, the medicine didn't make any problems for your granny's memory. So don't be afraid to use those simple anxiolytics, at least for now, when you need them so badly. There's no point in making your life difficult.

Dealing with that sort of insomnia, which is the most difficult, will have a twofold target. First, that the patient will sleep well, taking a powerful sleeping pill, which is to say a sedative of great effectiveness, but with a short period of life in the body, so that there are no traces of drowsiness in the morning. Taking this of its own is in many cases sufficient to reassure the patient, so that the following night they will not be overcome with anxiety whether they will be able to sleep.

For those sleeping pills the advice is to take them rarely and only when indispensable. In fact, they should not be taken on a daily basis, for after a week or two of regular intake they are less effective. They ought to be on the bedside table of every person suffering from insomnia, so that they can be sure that if necessary the problem will be solved. They must however be taken with discrimination and only occasionally, not every night.

However, for most cases of insomnia a treatment of longer duration with anxiolytics is required, since what led to insomnia was not a passing problem but a permanent inability to control anxiety. Over–stimulation of the brain with numerous and thorny worries raises the level of alertness so that when we go to bed to sleep the brain cannot calm down for sleep to come naturally.

Many people have the bad habit of thinking over the day's problems when they go to bed as well as what is pending for the next day. It is true that at the hectic pace of life today it is for many people the only moment they are alone with themselves and can better think through their serious and in particular their personal problems. From the angle, however, of healthy sleep it is the worst habit. Instead of relaxing, the brain starts questioning, thus blocking the switch leading to sleep. The computer does not shut down, so as to do the necessary operations of maintenance. It continues working and, in fact with limited functional capacity.

It is a big mistake to try to solve problems at night, with a tired and 'overloaded' brain. Because, contrarily, in the morning, after its daily maintenance, our brain is not only 'running' better, it can come up with solutions that could not be found at night! When our brain's 'desktop' is full we seek solutions in programmes that are spread out before us, so that what often happens is that we recycle and ruminate the same questioning impasse. When on the contrary in the morning the 'desktop' is empty and our experiences classified, our brain has the capacity to pull out programmes and solutions from zero. That is to say that it can cast a fresh glance, as we say, on the problems, consequently with a greater chance of solving them.

This has often happened to me: to wake up in the morning with excellent ideas in my head. Ideas and thoughts that make me ask myself 'why didn't I think of this before?' I think it is the same for most people, which is why I urge those who suffer from insomnia, to put off solving their problems for the morning. '… The solution may then present itself like a brainwave, a revelation'.

What is needed when going to bed is to direct one's thoughts to something painless – in every sense of the word. To a thought from which, nothing is expected to be born. In my case, in autumn and winter, when I close my eyes I think of a particular ski run. I concentrate on my legs and look straight ahead… A few seconds later I am asleep. In the spring and summer I play another video in my head: I am swimming off a particular beach. I have my head under water and see the blue colour of the water…

Some of my patients have told me that with these suggestions of mine they have made a video of their favourite route. The result is excellent. The video takes the brain out of the demands of thoughts and leads to calm. It does not give the thought process problems to solve, instead drawing the attention to painless representations.

As insomnia is the most frequent symptom in psychiatry and the second most frequent in general medicine after pain, I shall give some practical advice below as to how to deal with it.

10 recommendations for those who suffer from insomnia

1. Close your eyes and think of something pleasant, a meaningless scenario, such as e.g. an enjoyable route. Focus on the images of the route. Your thoughts will now leave the problems that are on your mind.

2. Do not think of your problems when you go to bed. Remember the best solutions are to be found in the morning, when your brain is rested. At night all the brain can do is repeat the same ruminations, which results in your being stressed.

3. Turn the alarm clock back to front, so as not to see what time it is when waking in the night hours. That is a usual source of anxiety. "3 o'clock, we say and I haven't yet fallen asleep… 4 ½ hours before I have to get up to go to work… I shan't be able to sleep and tomorrow I'll be dragging my feet again…"

4. Avoid watching a thrilling film before going to bed. When closing your eyes you don't want to imagine you are the hero being chased by the Mafia!

5. Do not drink coffee, tea, soft drinks of the Cola sort or anything containing caffeine.

6. Avoid heavy meals that will make you feel bloated.

7. Alcohol, while in small quantities inducing sleep, if however too much is drunk, will provoke wakefulness.

8. What is often recommended: "If you can't go to sleep, get up and have a warm bath or some hot milk" is wrong. One should on the contrary not do anything that is not in our customary routine.

9. Sleep should be a routine operation, meaning the same sort of time schedule and following the same procedures.

10. When a sleep schedule is changed, our biological rhythms need a couple of days to adapt. That must not worry us, it is absolutely normal.

The environment of sleep

THERE IS a tall tree next to my house, a ficus that must be more than half a century old. A party is held there every afternoon. Dozens or rather hundreds of birds, starlings and sparrows forgather and twitter for hours at a time. I see them sitting on a branch and then going to another one. They are constantly changing place, as if each one was trying to find the best where to spend the night. A spot that will protect it from possible rain during the night, that is that will have a roof of leaves over it. But at the same time, it must also afford protection from a hungry cat, so the branch must not be too low down!

It is a fact that while asleep the brain disconnects from the surroundings. A sleeping animal is vulnerable to the dangers lurking in the environment. Every animal therefore finds or makes a safe place where to sleep.

The ideal place to sleep is safe, so that the brain may 'disconnect' safely without putting itself in danger of harm. If a person does not feel safe they will not relax and consequently be wakened by the slightest external disturbance. It is what is called a 'catnap', the light sleep of an unsure being with a lot of enemies.

Furthermore, for someone to relax they must ensure ideal conditions of temperature that will protect from the probable drop of temperature at night. Remember that during sleep even the function of the body's central heating system is under-operating.

Together with the right temperature, the ideal spot for sleep must ensure little humidity and, obviously, protection from precipitations. Also there must be no noise, loud or intrusive, that evidently brings alertness.

When you think that we spend about a third of our life sleeping, you will see why this chapter is so important. Just as we place our desk with care and have good quality seating, as carefully must we arrange our bedroom and bed.

All this is, of course, subjective and it must be borne in mind that man is an animal with incredible capacities and adaptability. Humans can sleep under rain and yet be kept awake by a dripping tap. Some can sleep out of doors and others cannot relax until they have locked doors and windows and activated the alarm! This is the beauty and complexity of what the brain gives the weak and unprotected animal we call a human being.

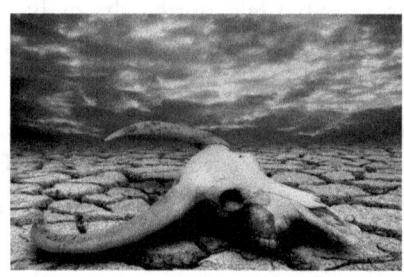

ANOREXIA NERVOSA

IT IS HIGHLY traumatic to lose something one has just gained. That phone call spelled for me one of my life's greatest disappointments: one morning I took a call from a colleague, the father of a 24 year–old student, to tell me his daughter had died two days ago. It was a knife stab to my soul. He was asking me, in a manner I could say was rather professional, unaffected by the tragedy, whether the medication with which I was treating her could cause low blood pressure. He was trying to find an explanation for the terrible event.

Three years ago his daughter had stopped her studies and was immured into a world where the only thing that interested her was food and calories. She spent most of her time at home, talking to her mother about diet and her thinness.

– *Shall I make you something to eat?*

– *No, I'll do it myself.*

– *But you haven't eaten anything since the morning.*

– *What do you know about it?*

– *Eat something or you'll die.*

– *I'm fine, I'll eat something at noon.*

— What will you have?

— That half apple I left in the fridge yesterday.

— But you can't live on half an apple.

— I also drink a pint of milk.

— And that's low fat too. How will you stay alive, my baby? You'll die. Your father is so worried... He wants to take you to hospital. He's a doctor and he knows. The way you are, you'll die. Your body is so weakened.

— Leave me alone, I know what I'm doing. And don't even think of putting me in hospital. I'll kill myself.

— But you are skin and bones. Can't you see it?

— I'm fine and there's nothing wrong with me.

It is true she looked like someone out of a Nazi concentration camp. Her blond hair had thinned, she had a light down on her face. She wore too many clothes because she felt cold and her periods had stopped two years earlier.

Conversations like the above were constantly repeated and if she did not speak, the same replies were signalled by her eyes every time her mother approached her. The mother with a look of pleading and the daughter with one of being sure: 'I know what I'm doing', 'leave me alone'. Like the power game played in puberty. Except that, in this case death was near.

When her father conquered his feelings of guilt and showed decisiveness, giving her the choice of either seeing a specialist or going to hospital, she agreed to visit me. Society has alas laden parents with feelings of guilt so, that they do not act effectively. Feeling guilty about the state their children are in, they allow things to evolve without doing anything about it.

The sweetest girl came to my office, showing from afar no trace of a problem. She was very skinny, true, but one sees so many thin girls in magazines and on TV. She was no less thin than the models on a catwalk. This one was much shorter in height, and that makes a difference in overall body mass, meaning the total quantity of fluids, because this little one was ultimately dying of dehydration.

It was when we shook hands that I saw the extent of the trouble. Her hand was skeletal, dry and downy and wrinkled. It was more the hand of an emaciated old woman than of a young girl. It had no vigour at all. The first thing that came into my head was an inner cry: "what a pity!"

She was reticent at first: I was after all her parents' choice and therefore their 'ally'. She was on the defensive, trying to persuade me that she was fine and had no problem. She maintained absolutely the master of herself, that it was something her mother wanted to deprive her of.

— *And what does your father say?*

— *He is influenced by my mother. She's the one who is hysterical about food. She won't leave me alone for a minute.*

— *And you, why do you stay there?*

— *Where should I go?*

— *Get your freedom. As you know, freedom is never given away for nothing. It's always conquered, usually at some cost. All you are doing is hurting your parents without yourself gaining anything. You prefer to shut yourself up in prison and slowly go to your death, rather than make a heroic exit, and happen what may.*

— *You mean leave home?*

— *Not easy, is it?*

Our terms gradually changed. Instead of being her parents' ally I was fomenting revolution, which she had evidently always wished for, but dared not. That way we forged a strong alliance that of course I must not betray. I became the ideal 'father', aligned against the mother, as well as the 'lover' who would elope with her, away from her family home. I tried to show her the way to independence: To finish college and leave home. I urged her to spread her wings and fly away. I showed her I trusted her, too, which she had missed so much. I realised I was the first person to believe in her capacity to fly on her own, without anybody's help. I said nothing about food. As if it did not exist. At some point she brought the subject up:

— *How can I stand my mother, when she's always chasing after me to eat?*

— *You'll have the target of freedom in front of you and that will give you the strength to be patient. Although you have to understand that it's reasonable for her, to worry about you. She has never seen you fly on your own and she's scared... But you must also know that you're playing with fire. You are so undernourished that you could easily die. That's why your parents are so worried, and rightly so... I know, you don't understand that. You feel you're normal, perhaps even that you're fat. That's the nature of the situation. Unfortunately you have gone beyond the limit of your organism and now you don't realise you're starving. There's a programme managing your brain that shields you from the pangs of hunger. That's also why your periods have stopped. Your body is economising on its faculties...*

— *But the first thing we need to do (using the first person plural on purpose) is to get rid of those assistance programmes... to be free again.*

— *But I don't feel I'm thin. How am I going to eat more?*

— *Now this is where I need you to help me. Try to eat more than you want, than your body wants. You'll manage gradually. Start with milk, let it be full fat. You can also add those powders to it with proteins and the necessary elements that add calories. Don't be afraid that you'll get fat. I'll give you some medicine that will not let your appetite grow. You'll take an antidepressant to lift your morale, because at the same time, as your morale is low, it reducing your appetite. Don't worry about losing control of your weight. I'll be keeping an eye on it and I promise I have the ways to keep you under control…*

It is the great anxiety of anorexics that they will lose control and go to the other extreme. In many cases it has happened in their past.

– …for my part, I'll do my best to make sure your parents do not force you to eat. I'll do everything I can to save you from their over–protectiveness, but, you have to be responsible for yourself. Please don't let me down.

When we had reached an agreement, I asked the parents to come and see me. I repeated what I had said to the girl and begged them to harden their heart and try not to pester her about eating and her intake of calories. It may be a risk, but there's nothing else to be done. The only alternative would be to hospitalise her daughter forcibly under prosecutor's order.

A month later the young woman came out of the house. She went back to her university courses, she saw her friends again. Her mother really did cooperate. The girl tried to increase her diet. The antidepressant had helped to get her going. I felt proud of her. Her parents began to relax.

As she was now revitalised, one weekend she decided to go with friends to a seaside resort near Athens. It was the first warm weekend, the first heat wave of this summer. That turned out to be her fatal mistake. The heat made the young girl sweat, she became dehydrated and she died suddenly. Nobody had thought of the heat wave and its consequences! Her father told me her friends had said that in the noonday heat the girl had opened the car door and tried to get out. She fainted and before anyone could do anything she was dead.

From heaven to hell! Everybody was stricken with grief and each one blamed themselves for what had happened: the mother, for her behaviour of rigorous over–protectiveness, and being locked in mother–daughter rivalry; the father, who albeit a doctor, had been slow to intervene forcefully for three years, and I, who with my optimism had had too much confidence in the girl. We had lost, all of us, but most of all, the 24 year–old student.

I have come across many other such patients in my career, young women, and men too, with anorexia nervosa, bulimia and other feeding disorders, mostly with a successful outcome. However, in developing the psycho–pathology and its treatment, always intensively involved are the personality of the patient, as well as relations with the parents and, above all, the models set by the particular society. This determining dependence on all those factors means that dealing with anorexia nervosa is a difficult matter and unfortunately it does lead some young girls to a biological death.

This fact gives the doctor much concern and he will search for the cause of such a tragic result: How is it possible for an intelligent and 'successful' young woman not to realise she is heading toward death? How can she not listen to the dramatic warnings, not only from her parents but also from the specialist physicians too and go to her death completely 'jubilant'?

Extreme anorexia: a programme for extreme situations

MY FIRST experience with anorexia nervosa as a psychiatrist was rather unorthodox. It was a young man and not woman as might be expected. He was very, very thin, like pictures from the Nazi Occupation in Athens. His weight was well below the 80% of his ideal weight for his height, but what was most surprising for the inexperienced doctor I was then, was that the patient was incapable of seeing how thin he was. He was an intelligent young man, with first class judgment and perceptions, who could pleasantly discuss all sorts of subjects of general interest, but as soon as his weight was mentioned, it was like talking to a wall. There was no way he could see that he was seriously underweight. So, although everyone around him had been seized with anguish about his future bodily health, fearing the worst, he faced the situation imperturbably which, if nothing else, was psycho–protection for himself.

I remember that we impatiently awaited the noon results of the bio–chemical tests, especially the levels of electrolytes, so as to give him intravenous serums and intra–intestinal nourishment. He, though, was on the contrary perfectly calm, was even surprised at our anxiety and attributed over–protective tendencies to us. It was also why he obstinately refused to be given serums and therefore this remained as our last resort of treatment – involuntary, it goes without saying.

Being so thin, one would expect him to fall on any foodstuff with special greediness. Instead, our patient felt full with the first mouthful of whatever dish. We used to say that his stomach was full and he felt satiated with a single chickpea from the delicious soup our hospital's cook served in those days!

At that time – the early 80s, the sector of psycho–endocrinology was in a phase of great blossoming. At our university psychiatric clinic we were conducting all the known endocrinological tests that could reveal even latent endocrinological disorders. It was therefore natural that in this case we should confirm what stood in the international bibliography regarding anorexia nervosa: the patient's endocrinal image was one of a male in pre–puberty, whereas his real age had passed puberty, years ago. Later we also found similar results in cases of women suffering from the disorder. Not only did emaciation suppress monthly courses, but also the woman's endocrine profile reverted to a pre–puberty level. And as is to be expected, a result of this hormonal regression is the suppression of any sexual urge in these patients.

Endocrinologists described this phenomenon as 'odd', a particularity of this specific illness. However, whoever has clinical experience of patients suffering from anorexia nervosa realises that the elimination of any sexuality is rather nature's protective 'foresight' for those patients and not a pathological symptom of illness. That is to say that nature, with effective prudence for those patients who have a minimum of calorie reserves, at the limit of biological death, suppresses any desire for the sexual act which, of course, normally leads to child bearing.

We have to bear in mind that the sexual act and child bearing are extremely important function – in fact a matter of survival – for animals. It has been observed that when an animal is in danger, or generally senses the approach of death, its sexuality automatically increases, as does its effort to have offspring. The ephemera, an insect that lives for only a day, for all 24 hours of its life seeks sexual companions in order to leave as many descendants as possible. In human beings this is seen in wartime, famine, natural disasters, even in great epidemics. Let us not forget that after World War II there was what is called the Baby Boom, an explosion of births. However, in the case of anorexia, nature seems to make an exception.

These observations led me to the conclusion that in patients suffering from anorexia nervosa, a special emergency programme is installed that tries to ensure the survival of the patient, reducing calorific loss to a minimum. Thus, not only is the sexual drive suppressed but so is the sexuality generally, provoking a regression of the entire mechanism of the hormones of the pituitary gland (hypophysis) that regulate the function of the gonads (ovaries and testicles).In anorexia nervosa the suppression of the sexuality is done centrally, from the hypothalamus and the pineal gland.

This suppression is radical and cannot easily be reversed. A sexual message, however strong, cannot reverse it. This means, it is useless to try to excite a patient with anorexia nervosa or try to trigger their desire for the other sex. They must first increase their weight above a crucial point for the pineal gland to begin functioning at the levels and rhythms of a mature person. Only then will they regain the capacity to be attracted and sexually aroused by the other sex.

The 'serenity' shown in sufferers of anorexia nervosa in the face of the danger to their life, as well as the total lack of the exceptionally unpleasant of feeling hungry, are evidently symptoms of a protective biological mechanism that operates in such situations. That is to say, I think there must be a mechanism in our brain for an emergency that enters into operation, in a state of undernourishment over a lengthy period.

When after a long time during which the organism receives fewer calories than it needs, the brain assumes there will not be nourishment available in the environment, so that for such patients the feeling of hunger is superfluous. As motivation, hunger cannot lead to an increase of the calories ingested, when food is not available. This means that hunger could only 'torment' the person, so the feeling of hunger in that situation is cancelled. In this way, subjects who do not eat as much as their biological sustenance requires, ceases to be tormented by hunger, since evidently there is no nourishment available around.

This was anyway valid until recently. That food should be at disposal but that a person will not, despite the hunger tormenting them, avail themselves of it is well known to be a 'perversion', due to social and psychological reasons and in our day is seen only in cases of anorexia nervosa.

The 'off–switch' which suppresses the feeling of hunger, appears to be in the all the animals' brain to serve in such exceptional circumstances, when although trying to find food impelled by their hunger, they can find none and are inevitably led to death from starvation. This is when the 'switch' goes 'off' and the person ceases suffering. Hunger is eliminated, they no longer feel weak, their body image alters and they do not see how thin they are. In this way they also cannot see the problem of their undernourishment nor the inevitable fatal outcome.

It is just this mechanism that, I think, gives that apathy the patients have, even when but a step away from death. It is a protective mechanism. It brings relief to people in extremely precarious situations, when undernourishment has reached a crucial and possibly irreversible point. The suppression of hunger and alteration of the body image bring elation to a person who Mother Nature thinks is going to die. They are offered an end without torment, leaving them with a misleading sensation of satisfaction, since they feel 'full' even if they have eaten only one chickpea, like my first patient with anorexia nervosa.

For the 'switch' to be 'on' again normally, that is for the person to be hungry again, there obviously first has to be weight gain. This means that the person has to be eating normally and have a positive calorie balance. Someone suffering from undernourishment must find sufficient food to be able to maintain themselves again and begin to gain weight, in order to begin feeling hungry again and be allowed to be conscious the extent of their weakness.

It is therefore quite useless to try to persuade an anorexic to eat. All we can hope for is that they should eat without being hungry, so as to increase body weight. Only then will they feel hunger and escape from their pre–death serenity.

Formulating this hypothesis helps on the one hand those who have to deal with cases of anorexia nervosa, to avoid useless quarrels with the patient. On the other hand it greatly helps the patients and their relatives, by giving a purely biological dimension to the problem. It removes the issue of over–protectiveness, always at the core of parent–patient relations. It even liberates the patients themselves who, simply because they were on a diet, were captured in the net of this 'protective' mechanism.

A slimming diet is uphill work and difficult in the beginning. But it becomes ever easier until later it turns into a slide downhill which, in fact in its final slope is very slippery and sometimes leads to death. Once someone is on that slippery slope, something drastic has to be done, otherwise, they will slip into death without realising it. The last stab of the knife is sweet and painless.

In any case, it has emerged that even when sufferers of psychogenic anorexia are able to restore their body weight, they can still relapse easily into the anorexic state. Indeed the level of difficulty of radical treatment depends on the length of time the patient had been underweight and malnourished. The longer their body operates under the protective program of the inhibition of hunger, the easier it is for the patient to relapse.

In other words, as the period of anorexia is extended, patients enjoy their extremely low body weight and become accustomed to their reduced food intake, so despite the fact that they are able to return to a healthy weight, they have already developed the 'bad habit' of consuming less than the minimum amount of food, which can often be far fewer than the necessary number of calories needed to maintain a healthy body. Indeed once patients become accustomed to the bliss they feel from minimal eating, they seek to return to the state of malnutrition. This explains the many relapses of the anorexic patient.

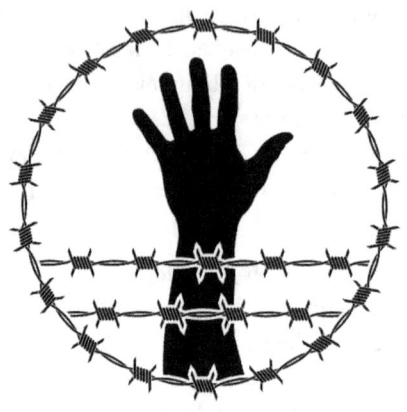

RESTRAINT

IN A WORLD of scarcity, as it is in the environment in which most wild animals and many human beings live, there is no reason to exercise restraint. Whenever they find food, they eat as much as they can, because they do not know what tomorrow holds. In times when nourishment is abundant, in fact, most animals store calories in the form of body fat. Fat has nine times more calories per unit of weight that proteins and hydrocarbons. The creation of fat stores was a great moment in evolution, since fat permits the animal to survive even when they cannot find food on a daily basis.

For wild animals the notion of restraint is absolutely useless. As long as there is food, they eat. If they find a mate they will copulate, so as to multiply and preserve the species. There is moreover a significant factor in the sexual act that makes it more difficult. In the name of evolution, nature requires that the female chooses the best male with whom to cross her genes. Better offspring will result from such cross–breeding. In sex, consequently, it is not restraint that is wanted, it is selectivity.

As this is the predominant notion in sexual functioning, why should it not be so in nourishment? Indeed, the only thing the animal requires is that; its food should not be poisonous and its drinking water should be pure. In this, it is usually assisted by its senses such as smell and taste. Therefore, the basic instinct of animals and, until recently of humans, was selection.

On the other hand, for humans, restraint was a totally useless faculty. Only religious teaching had promoted its usefulness, for it served to test the depth of the belief of the faithful.

But recently, thanks to brain power, Man was able to gather more food than was necessary for survival. Stores of fat fill up and up, grow, until in the end they are a threat to life itself. It is well known nowadays that too much food kills. We have reached the other extreme: whilst in the whole animal kingdom what kills is destitution, the lack of food and water, for some modern over–consumerist people, it is abundance that destroys.

The more hamburgers produced by fast–fooderies, the more they will try, through modern promotion strategies, to persuade us to consume them. The same goes for alcoholic drinks, cigarettes as well as narcotics. The more cheap products are available on the market, the more probability there is that our children too will become addicted.

In affluent regions of our planet therefore, modern man has to acquire the characteristic of restraint. It will save their life. And certainly restraint is a trait that should be cultivated from an early age, from even before school age. The sooner a child can control the need to consume, the better they will be able to defend themselves against the storm of message they will receive later.

Parents must be aware of the sort of world they are launching their children into. It is a world full of challenges; nightmare challenges, that easily drive one to the hunt for over–consumption. On the contrary, as the economy of our society is oriented toward over–consumption, anybody unable to join in the mad chase feels deeply disappointed.

I see cars capable of going faster than 200 km/hr and I feel inferior because mine doesn't reach 180. However, when I am discouraged by my inability to afford a fast car, something self–evident escapes me: that in any case I could not go faster than 130km/hr anywhere, since that is the speed limit on highways!

You can see how advertising has made us all run after imaginary needs. Needs our over–consumerist society has cleverly cultivated in us. Imaginary or bogus needs which, if we cannot satisfy them, may even lead us to depression.

On the other hand, fashion and social pressure to consume ever more, does often lead to comical situations too. Molière skilfully depicted the problem in his Bourgeios Gentilhomme (The Bourgeois Gentleman). I know a number of people who own luxury yachts, because that is what their social status requires.

The funny thing is many of them are seasick while still in the harbour! A lot of our purchases, that is, satisfy needs that are not real needs, they have to do with the codes of one's reputation in society.

I wear a watch that is very expensive because it withstands pressure in deep waters, especially designed for divers. I am proud to wear it and people comment to me about it. I admit I saved up quite a bit to be able to buy it although, I know perfectly well that because of an ear problem, I cannot dive deeper than two metres! So a simple cheap waterproof watch would have more than sufficed. What was it then that made me work harder to wear this marvel of technology on my wrist?

The answer lies in the codes given to us by society, in our course to achieve personal repute. It is in essence a game of fictitious reality, which, however, manages to mobilise our entire active society. Very few members of our society keep out of the game, and our society marginalises them. When you belong in the frame of society you are obliged to play by its rules.

The game is not an evil one. Besides, all progress and evolution is based on it. Without it we would stagnate, there would be no development of society. Money would not change hands. The rich would remain rich and the poor would live with they have. They would make no effort to go up in the world.

However, important as the game may be, what one must never let out of mind is that in a society of prosperity it is but a game of virtual reality. We must on no account allow it to stress us or depress us, if we have not achieved the objectives – which we ourselves, by the way, have set for ourselves.

My best friend was a very successful stock broker. At a time when the market was booming, he sold his firm and made an enormous amount of money. We had talks together and he would tell me about his plans to found a bank. From some comparisons he made, I gathered that for many years he had been in competition with a well–known banker. Moreover, I realised that in his fever to surpass this banker he was prepared to risk his every penny! For my friend it seemed perfectly natural to run a risk, if one were to be the winner. Of course, this was incidentally the key characteristic that led him to his phenomenal financial success. To me, his conservative friend, such a thing seemed outrageous. He spoke with passion about the millions he would make and which evidently would be more than his 'competitor'. Definitely, the figures he mentioned were out of this world for me. They belonged in the sphere of fantasy. I could not even see them as a subject to spend thought on: for me, there was little difference between ten or twenty million. Or even between ten or thirty million Euro.

But for my friend there was a difference because he had given himself the target of surpassing his 'competitor'. He had to do everything in his power to go over the limit of hundreds of million, which he himself had set as his immediate goal. There was a point when he reminded me of the businessman the Petit Prince had met. My friend was calculating, adding and multiplying numbers without the slightest interest in what they represented. So I said to him:

— *Listen here, my friend. I am a successful doctor and I may say I'm well off. So, I have ten pair of sunglasses at home. I've been buying them for years, either because I saw some with a design I liked, or when I was in an airport with time to kill and was trying one on somebody said they suited me, or because I was somewhere when I had forgotten my own. Thinking about that now, I may have more of them. But I wear only one, or perhaps two. The others just sit in a drawer.*

— *What are you getting at?*

— *You are wealthier than I am, you might have a hundred glasses. If your investment in your bank succeeds you may be able to acquire 1,000 or 2,000 sunglasses. And yet you, like myself, will use one or two.*

— *And that's a reason to have only two?*

— *No, of course not. But you must think that you will have no reason to use all the rest. I mean that today you have so much money it's enough not only to live in comfort for the rest of your days but that you can also ensure the same for your children and grandchildren when they come along. I don't mean you should stop work, God forbid, but don't you too have the right to enjoy what you have amassed?*

— *Yes that's true, I do have the right.*

— *You're chasing a figment of your mind. That you have 1,000 sunglasses and your competitor has 1,800. And both of you are working yourself to the bone to prove that one is better than the other...*

That was the last serious conversation we had. My friend did found his bank, but that summer was the first when he went on a relaxing holiday on his yacht with the company he really liked to have. He did not have a party for clients as he used to. Nor did he go to the jet set harbours to make an impression with his latest model of a boat. He was happy, in the true sense of the word. Playing no games so as to impress and promote his image. At last he had understood that he no longer needed to prove anything to anybody. He spent time on himself.

But unfortunately God sometimes plays his own tricky game with us his pawns. When he came back from his holiday he presented symptoms of lung cancer, although he had never smoked! He went to the biggest hospitals. He had chemotherapy and radiation, but nothing cured the cancer. He died within the year... just when he was beginning to enjoy life. It took many years for his wife, his children and his creditors to share out the 'thousands of sunglasses' he had left.

And I, when I had got over my grief, from now on every day I see the day as something gained. My friend and I were the same age, I was a few months the elder. In fact I remember that when we were little children he, with his business acumen, had 'persuaded' me into a contract that whoever died first was to leave the other his toys. When we shook hands on it, like grown-ups, he thought he had the better of me, since he was younger!

Not only is the dawning of a new day a day gained, but every day I try to enjoy my 'sunglasses' in the drawer as much as possible. I try to give them meaning, to enjoy them, to admire my face wearing them and not just count them in the drawer. I try to enjoy every Euro I earn, every word I say and everything I do.

Addictions: stuck in a useless programme

WE HAVE all experienced the fashion of the 90s, of the portable electronic games such as the well-known 'Game Boy'. In those days, everywhere you went you saw children, and adults too, absorbed by the game. They were fully concentrated, trying to arrange the geometrical shapes that came down from the top on the little screen of the toy contraption. I think that was the first game that conquered the hearts – or rather grabbed the time – of young and old, the well-known Tetris.

There was a lot of fighting over the game. Children fought over whose turn it was and of course, once begun they would not stop. Parents were unable to stop their children from spending their time on it. It was such a strong attraction that it was difficult for a sensible person to explain it.

At first the game made you anxious, as the new shapes to be arranged appeared. A little later it gave satisfaction when you had managed to make a row of shapes. This relaxed you temporarily, calmed you down. Then the stress returned as new shapes came up. If you saw the game coolly you could see that the challenge was ridiculous. Someone was worrying about arranging shapes on the screen of a toy machine! Yet most people could not desist. They could not ignore the challenge. They were not crazy, they were perfectly aware of reality and how ridiculous their action was. But they could not resist and refrain from it.

This is precisely what happens in addiction, whether it is compulsive gambling at cards or a general hunt for luck, even the sexual content of some addictions (fetishism, voyeurism, paedophilia, etc.). They are mental games some people feel compelled to play, or else they will be anxious. They know that most cases are destructive, but cannot stay away. They have to play for only then will they relieve the anxiety.

The secret in all those addictions is in the stress inherent in them and the relief from it they offer. In the unfolding of all those 'games' there are repeated points where dilemmas–challenges await the player. If the player 'gives the right reply' they will receive a confirmation in the form of a reward. Thus, the game stimulates the circuit of reward that is most probably in the brain's amygdale. It results in the player finding satisfaction in the game and wanting to continue, hoping for more satisfaction. So despite the appeals of logic that tell them to leave the game, the periodic stimulations of the reward circuit keep them at it.

Primitive hunter–man set traps to catch animals in order to survive. Usually a number of hunters got together to set the traps. However, from the time money and commerce came to an organised human society, man sets traps for money and the treasure troves of other fellow humans. Modern man therefore has two goals:

• On the one hand how to gain goods, either obtaining them through working or setting traps for others so as to take their goods.

• On the other hand, how to avoid falling into the traps others have constantly been setting for them.

One must be conscious of this double struggle. It must be kept in mind at all times that the course of life is full of traps. And predominantly, that it is very difficult to free oneself from a trap, once caught in one. It is therefore preferable to avoid them beforehand, rather than try to escape later.

It is preferable not to start smoking, rather than try to quit later. Better not go to a casino, than to try later to disentangle oneself from the net, having lost both money and dignity. Most traps are so well designed as to make the struggle to liberate oneself seems pointless.

I once had a patient, who had lost a fortune at cards and casinos. He had reached the point of being hassled by money–lenders and getting beaten up. Since it was not possible to restrain him from going to the casino, I urged him to leave Athens and go and live in his home town where there was no casino. There he married and had a family, but when three years later he came to Athens on a visit, he made sure to find a hotel room from the balcony of which he could see the Mt Parnes Casino of Athens!

–If I can't go… At least I can see it, Doctor.

It often happens besides that people are sent to jail for sexual crimes such as child pornography and who, when they are released and although they know that if they continue they will re–arrested, cannot resist their obsession. Once a person's mind is caught in such traps it is, unfortunately, not possible to escape.

This is why the fight has to focus on avoiding the traps. The young must be taught how not to be influenced by all that enticing advertising of all those traps. They must take pleasure from uncovering a trap and avoiding it. Let us teach them to feel like a soldier on landmine clearance, who is happy whenever he finds a mine. For those charming and seemingly innocent games are a mine laid in the life of youngsters: from narcotics to computerised games.

An innocent game of strategy

ONE DAY a couple, friends of mine, came to see me.

— *We need to talk to you. We have a big family problem with our son.*

— *What's the matter, why are you so upset?*

— *Our son spends more and more time at his computer.*

The wife replied, who was more talkative and decisive than the husband. It is worth noting that it has been see that in most couples, it is the wife who takes the initiatives. It is she who spurs the man, whether to move house, take a holiday or leave the parental home where they are cohabiting. In this instance it was the lady who decided, they should come to see me and ask my opinion about their son's addiction.

Their son, Alexander, was then about 35 years old, married to a dynamic young woman who, before becoming pregnant and having their child had worked in a public relations firm. The child is now two and they live independently in a flat above my friends'. It is an elegant two–storey building in a seaside suburb of Athens. My woman friend has plenty of time to spend with her grandson. The front doors of both flats are open practically all the time. The daughter–in–law and the boy spend more time at the grandparents' than in their own flat.

Alexander, the one with a problem with the computer, had studied architecture. He works in a technical office he has opened with a friend. Their last project was a block of flats in an urban quarter. In the past year, because of the economic building slump, the office does not have much work and both partners are under–occupied.

— *Alexander spends more than ten hours a day playing games on the computer.*

— *Strategy games?*

— *How should I know? All I can tell you is that he says he builds towers and castles and has a team that attacks others and they conquer spaces. I don't know what to say. I think it's laughable. He's a professional and he occupies himself with such things...*

— *Don't say that.* I answered. *I'm afraid that sadly, quite a lot of my patients have become entangled in games like that of virtual reality. In virtual reality they can choose a personality,* be Zorro or Superman and perform heroic feats. *In virtual reality they escape from the harsh reality which for most of them is miserable and with no way out. I think that's why these games are so popular.*

— *What do you mean?*

— *When you take the personality, or rather, when you enter a persona of a tall, handsome and powerful hero, you identify with him. While you're playing and are in the virtual world of heroes, you feel one of them. You forget you're short and ugly, poor, and above all cowardly and frightened. In the virtual world, at no cost, you are fearless, unless you're playing for money. But even then, you're only losing money, you're not being beaten or injured, nor is there any danger of being killed. You lose fictitious lives. That is besides a casino's philosophy. It's a luxurious place and when you enter it, you feel you too are part of this opulence. I remember the first time I went to the casino in Monte Carlo I thought I was a lord, even though I was only a poor tourist. Although I am conservative by nature, there I began to take risks. In fact, when I won something, meaning my risky behaviour was rewarded, I became bolder until of course I lost all my winnings. That's how the system is organised. To reward you every so often, so that you keep on daring.*

— *What about Alexander? What reward does he get in this game of strategy?*

— *When you win points you don't only get the virtual reward from the game itself, such as forts and a virtual area, you are also rewarded by the friends who are playing with you. Just as in football, when you place a goal, you gain the esteem of your team and you also gain the cheers of the crowd in the tiers.*

— *Do you mean you think his wife is proud of him? Well, I can tell you, she isn't. On the contrary, she complains and grumbles all the time... He's at that computer for more than ten hours a day. His wife suggests a walk with the child and he won't go. He urges to go out alone, because he's always at 'a crucial stage' of the game. We often wonder how she stands it. The way he's behaving he'll make her either leave him or find a lover. And I, his mother, declare that she'll be absolutely justified if she does.*

— *And at the same time, he feels he's a winner, riding his horse!*

— *It's very serious doc... What we mind about is his son. My grandson is at an age now when he begins to understand. It's not just that his father doesn't spend time with him, doesn't play with him nor takes him for a walk. It's that he sees his father at the computer all the time. What sort of a model will the boy have?*

— *You do have a point. He sees a wanker...*

I used a strong word on purpose, to shock them. When I think I have reached my target I throw in, something particularly provocative. Only what hurts can bring forth some alteration. Kindness does not bring a change. It can only bring relaxation and a repetition of the mistake.

I went on to say:

— *The virtual reality game is exactly like masturbating. In his fantasy the masturbator can have and make love to any babe he calls to mind, with no trouble and without risking rejection. Safe in his room he chooses whichever woman he wants ... Of course, life goes on outside.*

— *And that's just why we want your opinion. How we should deal with it. We know it's serious and we wanted a specialist's view. What should we say to Alexander and what to his wife?*

— *Exactly what I said to you. Use the comparison with the masturbator. It will shock him and is the only thing that can get him away from his computer. I'm afraid all the other things you will have said to him don't work: "it isn't right to spend so many hours at it", "give some of your time to your wife and child" ...only the social stigma of masturbation and the insulting 'wanker' can get to him. There is no excuse for masturbation. Isn't it the same with smoking? Anything one can say about cancer and heart disease doesn't count. Only the social ostracism of smoking and smokers can make them quit the habit. The mere fact that they are banished out of doors and that they are regarded as being tainted really helps them quit their harmful habit. In societies where smokers are seen with kindness and forgiveness, as being persecuted, smoking will not diminish.*

— *So what do we have to do?*

— *It would be better for his father to speak to him and tell him that what he is doing is masturbating. Then handle him in the same sense, that is, substitute the word masturbation for 'playing'. When he says he's going to his room to play, tell him he's going to masturbate. Tell your daughter–in–law to say the same. Have her confront him with the label of masturbator. Let her entice him into reality, that is, to be sexier while at the same time sneering at masturbation.*

Following this brief conversation, I saw them again a few months later. They told me they had put off applying my drastic strategy at first, but that later they were forced to do, because things were getting worse. In the end they admitted, I had been right. They all had to become more crude, even his wife, who said she felt humiliated by his 'masturbating'. Only then did he get it and completely stop playing computer games.

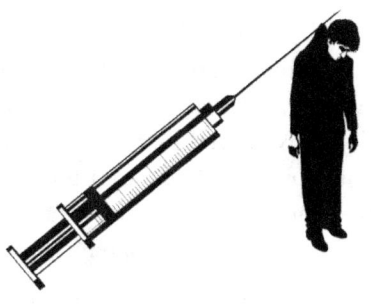

NARCOTICS

I COULD not avoid becoming involved in this major problem, since I practice psychiatry. Of course I do everything possible to keep my distance from users, but the continuous spread of illegal use of narcotics unavoidably brings me in contact with parents on the one hand, who ask me for my advice and on the other with 'specialists' who trumpet diverse theories, as to the solution of the problem.

What I try to do for the first category is to rid them of guilt. Parents nowadays feel responsible for every wrong–doing of their children. In modern Westernised society, in that sense, if a child fails its exams, in its school or university studies or does not reach its objectives, it is mainly the parents who are socially humiliated and not the student who doesn't care. They feel guilty in case they did not make sure that their offspring went to tutorial school with the best tutors, or enroll them in the best school, or oversee their homework, or did not serve a good home–cooked meal when they were sitting their exams.

The same thing happens when it becomes known that some young person is taking drugs. The parents immediately feel guilty. They wonder what they did wrong in their upbringing. As is naturally to be expected they start blaming one another, leaving out the principal offender, who is none other than the user himself.

The story generally begins with the mother finding traces of hash or other substances. Remains of grass in the child's pocket or bag, frequenting 'suspicious' friends, odd communication, spending a lot of time closed up in a room with friends, or even finding cash missing. There may also be a change of behaviour.

Not that any of that may be exclusively attributed to the habituation of the young person to narcotics. They could all easily be attributed to puberty or also to the desire of the young to be liberated.

This is also always the parents' excuse for what they found but could not believe. Aside from the natural denial, the first psychological reaction to the terrible, literally, 'suspicions', what reinforces the mother's 'silence' is the guilt she feels at the bottom of her soul. If she told the father about them, the first thing he would do would be to blame her. This usually triggers a to–and–fro of reactions and accusations as to who of the parents is more to blame.

In fact, if it should happen that at the time of the discovery the parents are separated, the guilt is immediately shouldered by whichever was responsible for the separation. This contemporary social myth, that the children of a split family are more susceptible to every form of offense and in consequence also drug use, is nowadays the prevailing ideology of our times.

The roots of that myth lie in the days when narcotics were scarce and difficult to find. A generation ago, when drug use was really a habit acquired by unhappy people who needed relief from their mental trouble, or by young people looking for new sensations, it could have been said that the family ambience could have played a role in the entanglement of the young in narcotics.

Today, sadly, the reality is very different. There is an abundance of narcotics, resulting in everybody being the target of a cleverly planned and particularly aggressive traffic. There are no longer any vulnerable groups to become potentially susceptible targets, nor of course are young people protected by a family warmth or close family ties.

— *So, Doctor, there isn't anything we can do to protect our child? I can't believe there is no way to prevent it...*

A panicked mother told me, who came with her husband to consult me, because narcotics were found in their daughter's class.

— *The only thing you can do is try to keep your daughter from being a target. This means she shouldn't show her financial ease and especially that she does not have a lot of money at disposal. Not go around with more pocket money than what she needs for the bare necessities, and that too strictly controlled. Give her what she spends a day without extravagance, or rather impose restrictions. If she wants to buy an article of clothing, give her exactly as much as she* asks for and obviously ask to see the receipt. Children with plenty of money are the favourite targets for drug traffickers.

— And her friends?

— She may be offered drugs by the most angelic of persons. It could even be a friend of hers from a family you know, who is 'above all suspicion'. I would tell you in fact to beware of just such people, because affluent families are the traffickers' top target.

They looked at one another, at a loss, trying to assess their daughter's girlfriends one by one.

— You should also know that if a user manages to bring in another two or three as customers, they might get their own fix for free. Therefore, anybody might try to involve your daughter in the racket. They needn't be a dealer or a chronic addict. That's for TV. Your daughter is in no danger from Escobar the coke king, but she could be from her girlfriend Nana.

— What can we tell her to protect her?

— Just what I said to you. Also, that she shouldn't feel ashamed of not smoking hash, nor that she is a stick–in–the–mud. On the contrary, nowadays it's ultra–fashionable to be able to refuse. She should say thanks and leave the place where they are using. Warn her too that some people could have pretended to be buying only to infiltrate places where narcotics circulate under cover for the police. And that others got involved merely because their friend had some narcotic in his pocket… And that "it's an awful pity to have a police record and not to be able to find a job in the future, just to be 'with it' or worse, to cover a friend." That's what you should say. Don't be over–dramatic with prohibitions and over–protective exaggerations… Just be a friend.

— But what you're saying is terrible.

— And yet, if you go over the top and express horror, all you'll achieve is that your warnings will be ignored or even impel her in the opposite direction from what you want. Never forget that young people are very curious, so that if you tell her about disastrous side–effects and satanic friends who will try to exploit her, you may very well arouse her fantasies. Quite a lot of the young become involved merely because they want to prove to themselves or somebody else that they can handle difficult situations and that they can 'resist' the effect and side–effects of drugs, just as they do with alcohol, to show how tough they are!

— But that's so hard. It's like walking in a mine–field to talk about drugs but calmly and coolly… How is it possible to talk about such a frightful subject without being vehement?

— Just as you would about driving. It isn't you, who forbid her to drive a car, but the law says you can get a permit from the age of 18 when you pass a test. If you impose a prohibition in your relationship, you may expect that she will try to get around it. It's the same for narcotics. It's better not to show you are panicked and that it's your weak point. It's preferable in fact, in view of the repercussions, to refer rather indifferently to third parties, not to say "Watch out, you'll be arrested", but "I have a colleague, the poor man is living a nightmare: they caught his *son smoking pot with a friend and is running around to lawyers, to the police and jail to get him out."*

A parent's task is a difficult one, for it is believed nowadays that everything has to be done, in every way, to shield one's children from any danger. The idea is absolutely narcissistic and goes hand in hand with a feeling omnipotent. It is unfortunately difficult for a parent to admit the limited capacities they have. In any case, the young today are more influenced by the Media, the Internet, friends and school. Parents, like teachers, can exert more influence by setting an example than by warnings and counsels.

There is also something else, equally hard but totally realistic, especially in regard to narcotics. When a family is carried away by a torrent, parents try to save as many children as they can. Those that cannot be saved are let go, so that not everyone drowns.

Alas, the world of narcotics is pitiless. If someone becomes entangled in its web, it is extremely difficult to escape. Initially it is because they delude themselves that it can be controlled.

– As for me, Doctor, I can quit whenever I want to. It's up to me… I just enjoy it… and that's why I do it.

There is no greater deception than that. There is unfortunately no way to resist the temptation, after repeated experience of drug use that energise the brain and give a fleeting sensation of euphoria. It is natural that they should want to repeat this voluptuous feeling. In fact, as time goes on the interval between having the effects of the substance seems ever more miserable and finally unbearable, so that the result is of course to try in every way and at any cost, to make sure of the next fix.

My experience has shown that there are two ways of stopping this downfall:

Either because at the outset there was a heavy price to pay for the consequences of the habit, if for instance they have the good luck to be caught by the police and get into bad trouble, or if family and friends react excessively as soon as it is known that they are embroiled in drug use.

The other crucial point is when the user feels intense humiliation. If the phrase goes through their mind of: "look at what I have become… and I'm stealing from my mother, or… mobile phones from little kids, or even… that I'm selling my body to get my dose". If the feeling of shame is activated before it is suppressed by long habit, it is the final point where there is hope of a real escape from the slippery slope.

Most people may find these words particularly pessimistic, but they are sadly more true than the facile hopes on which another deal is based: the hope of a 'detoxification' or 'rehab'. All I can do is devalue those 'specialists' who every so often intervene from some platform of the media to suggest solutions.

The issue of narcotics is purely a social one. It is the same as smoking and traffic accidents. It is neither a medical issue nor of upbringing. The facts are indisputable:

Smoking and heart attacks resulting from it are diminished only, wherever anti–smoking laws are in force. Information campaigns against smoking and the medication that helps to quit, have very little effect. It goes for traffic accidents too. They are less only where there is strict police control. The very same 'dangerous drivers', when they are driving in countries with strict rules, automatically become the safest and most polite drivers, simply from awareness that laws are enforced there.

It is not a theoretical position, nor a working hypothesis, as is the much–discussed scenario of legalisation which is supposed to free users from the dealers: there where the legal system is harsh, as in Singapore, drug use and dealing have been practically eradicated. It is only in such an environment, that our children might not be in any danger from narcotics and their consequences. No other theory has unfortunately been proven to be effective, wherever in the world it was applied.

Conforming is achieved only by control. This is because human nature fortunately, has the inclination to try to surpass the limits imposed. It is the same impulse that led mankind out of caves to reach this point. On the way, of course, some were destroyed because they attempted... poisoned fruits that looked so pretty. Whoever of the remainder of the people was intelligent observed what happened to them and avoided tasting the enticing fruits, and life and evolution continues because of them.

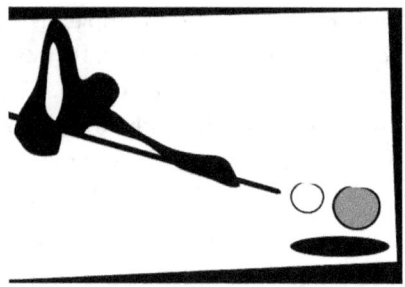

PROVOCATIVE PSYCHOTHERAPY

IN HIGH school, although mine was a very good school, I was a middling student. I often did my homework in the break before a class and was generally more interested in extra–curricular activities: parties, girls, scooters, tennis and so on. I was not interested in competing with my schoolmates who sat in the front row, who had always already prepared the next subject matter so as to show the teacher, that were all–knowing. As for me, whenever a teacher had me sit in the front row, it was because I was chatting or giggling with my neighbours at the desks. It was therefore no surprise that when sat the admission exam for medical school I failed miserably.

I was vastly disappointed and so were my parents, who clearly expected better results. Nevertheless, however, my relatives and friends all said "Never mind. You'll study harder and try again next year", or, "a lot failed who had studied very hard", or even "it's a question of luck too. Next year you'll have more luck". These are the comforting words usually heard after a failure, which are meant not to discourage the person who failed in their attempt. Trying, that is, to encourage, giving excuses for the failure.

But one morning I was walking down one of the main central avenues of Athens and came across a schoolmate, one of those who usually sat in the front row. He stopped me and asked if I had passed the entrance exams of medical school. When I said I hadn't, he preened like a peacock and said something I shall never forget: "It's only what you deserve, you and the other yobbos... I came near top for the Athens Philosophy School!"

I felt like I had been struck by a thunderbolt. I hadn't expected it. It was the absolute opposite of everything that had been said to me until then. It gave me a shock. And then something fundamental changed inside me. I was so ashamed that it transmuted to determination. Determination to succeed and show everyone that I was no yobbo.

Honestly, my life changed from that moment on. Not only did I study assiduously and pass the exams for the Athens Medical School the next year, I got such high marks that I was amongst the first at the top. I was totally transformed and it continued. I passed all the exams at the first go with top marks.

My new identity, of the hard-working, diligent and studious persona has stayed with me ever since. I graduated with no delays and I still feel guilty when I am lazing around without doing anything productive.

Ever since, I feel deeply grateful to my old schoolmate who attacked me so nastily when we met at that spot. Were it not for that I might still have been contending with the forces that kept me complacent and mediocre. His cutting remark provoked my psychological reaction. It shook me and showed me a reality, I did not want to face. I have to say that the comforting words of my friends and relatives were just providing me with the excuses that I wanted, to continue in my life on the same lines. The excuses did not impel me to turn the page. They were much too convenient to allow me to go on as I was, making the same mistakes without losing out psychologically.

As for my revenge, which at that critical time of my life I promised myself I would have, it came decades later. It was at a reunion of old schoolmates in a restaurant in the northern suburbs. I recognised him in spite of the number of years that had gone by. I went up to him and asked him about his career, as is usual at such gatherings. He told me that when he graduated from the School of Philosophy he had been appointed a high school teacher, first in the provinces and for the past years he taught Ancient and Modern Greek and History in a high school in Athens.

It was obvious he did not remember the incident that had changed my life. He asked me about my career and I told him, without any sign of boastfulness in my expression nor my tone of voice, very simply that I was teaching Psychiatry at the Athens School of Medicine.

This story motivated me, to form my personal strategy in the way I deal with those who ask me for psychiatric help.

First of all I realised that a word or an event can have dramatic repercussions in the course of a person's life. It is not an effort in vain to intervene in the programme set up in their brain. It is not necessary to spend hours, days, months and years, as classical psychiatry teaches, to achieve the desired changes in a person's programmed behaviour. An appropriate, acute and above all well–timed strike may be sufficient to change the course of someone's individual history.

Looking around us we can see many examples of events that changed the character, the personality of people we know. Rejections, separations, deaths, disasters… What is odd is that unpleasant events can better change us, than the pleasant ones. So many people won the lottery of happiness but in themselves stayed wretched and poor well–timed; while on the other hand rich people who for some reason 'lost everything', when once they had got back on their feet, saw life differently.

It seems it is more of a shock, that is provokes a greater psychological shake–up when something negative occurs, than when it is positive. Evidently, in intensely negative situations self–protective mechanisms go to work that are very powerful in being able to modify programmes that are 'running' in the brain, with the ultimate objective always of a better survival for us.

Reward, contrarily, is not as intense in enabling a modification of the operational system of our mind. This is why it has been shown that punishment is more effective to change behaviour than praise. In experiments conducted by behaviour specialists with mice, punishment by electro–shock is a more successful way of teaching than the reward of sugar – as long of course as the animal is not hungry, whereupon the sugar is a means for survival. It is worth noting of course that these old conclusions of behaviourists, because they are not 'politically correct' since they propound punishment as a teaching tool, have fallen into disuse among 'progressive' psychologists.

Punishment in fact plays a role of virtual reality very often and is repeated in our mind every time we try to apply a forbidden and condemnable programme. That is the educational strength of punishment, which it would be wrong for the psychiatrist not to take advantage of, when he is in essence trying to change the behaviour pattern of the person, who has come to ask for it.

In consequence, an earth–shaking event or word that could activate self–protective forces, at a time when one's existence is at a difficult stage, may bring about a decisive change in the brain's programmes which we had so far been using.

This is how I started being provocative and 'aggressive' to some extent with my patients. I point out to them where they are wrong and indeed, I paint the most garish picture of what awaits them in the future, if they continue in the same behaviour that brought them so far.

A strike where it hurts

I TRY as a matter of fact, to have an attitude as provocative as possible, for it to have as much of an impact as possible. This is not difficult, for most people who come to a psychiatrist expecting to find an 'ally': Someone who will understand them and be on their side. Someone who will sympathise and, 'why not?' tell them they are right.

So many ask me from the start to meet together with their companion – if that is where the problem lies – believing implicitly that I, as a psychiatrist, will needless to say defend them. Others bring their parents along, who 'repress' them, believing I shall take their side and justify them.

How disappointed they are, when they hear me say that the problem is basically their own. Not of those who repress but, of their own for giving in without reacting.

A woman's voice on the phone urgently requests an appointment. She sounds very anxious and says she badly needs help because she has reached a point of desperation in her life. When I hear the word 'life' I pay special attention to the words that person uses. Of course I know it is nothing but a move to make an impression, a 'strong card' to put down on the table of transaction with the people around. It is however still an indication, that the person playing this 'card' is desperate. And there is no doubt at all that a desperate person is a person in danger. A desperate person is capable of anything and must have our attention.

This lady who wanted so urgently to see me also asked for an appointment "as late as possible… the last of the day" because she wanted her husband to come too and he worked late hours.

In my experience, there are usually two sorts of people who want to be accompanied: those who are having a panic attack and those who are 'quarrelling' with their companion. From her voice and what she said, I placed her in the second group.

I do like to play a guessing game of my own. To try to foretell what someone wants from me or what the illness is, based on the fewest possible elements. It is something that had made an impression on me, when clinical doctors of the old 'French school', as it was called, could make a diagnosis from experience at first sight of a patient.

So, when I heard this woman's voice, I said to myself that she had a problem with her husband and wanted to go to a professional to say she was in the right, gave her an appointment for the evening of the next day, and waited to be proved right too!

The next evening, then, I opened the door of my office and saw before me a lady 40 to 45 years old, elegantly dressed, with no nouveau–riche extravagance, although she was wearing a gold watch and had obligatory brand–named handbag. She was not some 'babe' but she was certainly attractive. The man who came in behind her was evidently the husband. A man of about sixty who showed clearly from his look and posture that he was there against his will. Even the way alone in which someone comes into the room may reveal quite a lot of elements. In this case, the woman practically shoved the door to come in, while the husband hesitated and took a little time, enough to insinuate that 'I don't want to be here… I'm doing it as a favour'.

I showed the lady into my office and asked the husband to take a seat in the waiting room. She reacted:

– *No, I want him to listen. Anyway, what I have to say concerns us both.*

I am firm on this point and make myself clear:

– *Don't worry; the gentleman will come in later. We will have all the time needed to discuss anything you want together.*

She came in and I closed the door. I showed her to the comfortable armchair on the other side of my desk and I went to my chair, whereupon I heard a stream of words:

– *You will have gathered that is my husband. We have been married ten years and I can't take it any longer. The cup is overflowing. My life is completely bogged down. He will not go out; he is absolutely cut off from me. We hardly talk at home. He says he's absorbed by his work. I feel neglected. I've reached the point of wondering if my life is worth living.*

In my office the armchair for the patient is at an angle as it is for the colleague in an office and you need to turn the torso to see the person behind the desk. While this lady had been talking, she had looked straight ahead as if she were addressing an invisible audience. When she stopped, she turned around and looked me straight in the eye. Her eyes were filled with tears.

So as to restrain the melodrama to which evidently the woman intended to lead us, I broke my silence and asked something that would put us back on track, which at least for me, initially was to find out what the "rules of the game" were.

– *Do you have children?* I asked.

– *Two. Two girls, nine and seven. But it's not the children who are the problem. They're good kids and I have to say their father loves them and spends more time with them than most fathers. The trouble is in my relationship with him. About me he doesn't care at all.*

– *So it's you who has the problem.* I observed.

—No, he's the one who has a problem. She said emphatically.

Now I was getting close to where I wanted: to 'hit' her where it hurt.

— But it's you, who came asking for help (stressing the 'you'). He didn't seem to be under stress. He's sitting out there and if we tell him to leave, it looks as though he'd be quite happy to.

It is a fact, that one can rarely realise the terms and the rules of the game we are playing. It is usual to think that everything moves, or ought to move, on the axis of our self. We think the movement of those around us is like the orbit of a satellite, just to give us light, meaning to be of use to us. We forget, however, that even in the case of the moon, when it does not cast light on the earth in an eclipse, it is the fault of the Earth that casts its shadow on the moon. In the same way it is our own fault, if a relationship no longer brings us what it used to in the past.

The most usual is gradually to marginalise our companion and at some point, to realise they are no longer shining as of old. It is easy to understand, from the description alone, that the mistake is not the companion's but our own, for allowing our relationship to develop in that way. The other, simply finds a role that satisfies his or her dreams and aspirations without provoking friction and clashes. This is how most relationships silently wear out.

I try to avoid the words 'wearing out' although they are those most used in the sector of relationships, because it suggests something inevitable, something normal. No, I do not believe that such as a scenario is inevitable. It is a normal development only if both sides do not try to maintain their relationship. It is unfortunately natural, if nothing is done, for the routes of two people who start out on a relation of companionship, to distance themselves gradually and to drift apart. For this not to happen, both have to make an effort, use up some energy. Bonds need energy to maintain their cohesion. One has to fight natural laws all the time. Just as to stand up we have to combat the laws of gravity, in the same way, to stay together we have to keep the other close energetically. Not passively. Not to react only to their stimulation but produce some stimulation ourselves, take initiative ourselves. From a compliment or a caress, to an unexpected gift, or a plan for a trip.

— I asked for help because I'm the weaker link in this marriage. This is not the way things were when we got married. I was his princess, he looked after me, we travelled… we had a good time… (Her face hardened.) *He gradually put me aside, he doesn't look after me. That's why I asked for your help, to show him my needs. That's why I brought him along, for you to talk to him. I can't bear it any more, I'm shattered.*

— You mean you want me to tell him to care for you more, because you're shattered. For the good of your health… And supposing he believes me and changes. This could be for a week, a

month… two months at most. Then he will let go and be again what he is now. Then you'll be back at square one, as you are now. Then what?

— *Well, what do you advise me to do? There's no other solution, I've tried everything.*

— *If as you say you've tried everything and have reached this point, there are two things you can do: either you come to terms that this is how he is and go on like this for the next 50 or 60 years you have ahead of you…*

— *Aren't you optimistic, Doctor!*

— *Why? We may all reach to be a hundred… at least.*

A smile escaped her.

It was what I needed to strike decisively.

— *… But if you don't like this precise prospect, you can separate. Nothing is keeping you anyway. As I understand, living with him has become a Calvary for you. Why stick with it?*

— *And what about the children? Do you think I haven't thought of that too? But it would be like killing my children.*

— *Why do you say that? You think people who divorced killed their children? Nowadays in our country one in three marriages ends in divorce. I don't think all the children that correspond to those divorces have any particular problems. Of course I'm not saying it's the best solution, but it must be hard to live like this for the next fifty years…*

The art is to keep a subtle balance. No way should one seem only nasty and aggressive. Strategic strikes are needed, successively on the nail and on the anvil. The philosophy is: I'm with you, so that together we can find what is best for you and what you are prepared to do and to give up from your best interest. Because one thing is certain and the patient must be convinced: that nothing can happen without an effort and sacrifices being made. No change happens of itself.

I try to find and to show the alternative propositions for life. I do not idealise these proposals in any way. I do not make the mistake that friends and relatives make, who idealise the directions that agree with their own personal beliefs. In cases such as the lady's, I had before me the parents usually say the couple should not part. On the other hand her divorcée friends invite her to join the club. I have even seen an instance where a 'friend', after having engineered her friend's divorce, took the ex–husband whom she had earlier been accusing!

The doctor has to have great self–knowledge and self–restraint, so as not to get involved and propose just anything. Even in what in some cases seems self–evident, the doctor must not in the least allow it to show that he proposes it. I am not saying that I often want to utter my opinion spontaneously. What any third person would express in my position, whether a friend or a relative: an obvious view that could be based for example on a manifest disharmony between the couple, or the character, or social status, or upbringing, or the age or, finally, the physical appearance of the two sides. However, although this might at first seem to flatter one of the sides and reinforce the doctor's relation with them, it would in essence cancel the doctor's role. It would place him in the position of any friend, relative or third person.

One should, besides, at all times be aware that a patient will usually see the psychiatrist as an alternative solution to their problem and therefore 'court him/her' or flirt, either openly or insinuating in a hidden way. It is therefore very easy for the psychiatrist to be drawn into the game, particularly when the other is an interesting person of the opposite sex. That way he will however lose his objectivity and it will be as disastrous for the patient who asked for help, as for the doctor.

The first and optimum attribute of a psychiatrist is not knowledge but restraint, self–control and self–knowledge that must always be exercised in the practice of psychiatry. They must always be aware of what 'the game' is between them, the patient and eventual third parties involved (spouses, parents, friends). I do not mean the sexual aspect alone, but it may happen that for instance the stance of a patient's parent may awaken memories of our own of parental oppression which without our realising it may turn one against the patient's parent, sometimes with harmful effect on the patient.

To revert to the case of the woman in question, what I do is to give a tragic aspect to both the alternatives. This is easier since, it does not entail the risk of prettifying the one that suits me best personally.

– You can of course go on living marginalised in your husband's life. He would be occupied with whatever occupies him now, while you will stew in your own juice... But tell me something: is your husband happy with his life?

– Yes of course. At least it looks like it. He doesn't complain any more.

– Oh, so he grumbled?

– Yes, when the first child was born he started grumbling. He wanted stuff I couldn't give him. At the time we had had quite a lot of problems in our relationship. In fact his parents had intervened. But then, after the second child was born he gradually quietened. He is relaxed and doesn't complain any more. He seems happy enough...

– With a new relationship?

– What are you saying, Doctor? My husband? He has never given any sign of... In any case that's out of the question because I didn't tell you..., he has a sexual problem.

– Does he not have sex with you?

– *That's right. For the past three years he's been impotent.*

– *With you?* (As the first time she did not get it, I had to be more precise.)

– *No, he can't be aroused generally. He has a problem.*

– *Is he diabetic, have MS, a bad heart problem, or does he take medicine that cause the problem?*

– *Nothing of all that. It has just happened gradually over the years. At first he wasn't in the mood and later when he tried he couldn't.*

– *With you?* (I insisted sounding teasing).

– *My husband is not like that...*

– *Like what? Do they have some special indication?*

– *He's a stay-at-home type. He likes the children. He doesn't like to go out... Anyway, he has no free time: he goes from home to work and work to home.*

– *So the 'other woman' is where he works.* (I said with an air of Hercule Poirot having just solved a case.)

– *Why are you insisting, Doctor?*

She had long not been looking so sad any more. She had become the tiger protecting her young or whatever she considered to be hers. Her claws were out and her voice had hardened. I was imperturbable, expressionless, not moving so much as an eyebrow, glad she had taken the bait. Whilst at the start, the husband was a satellite who was not of service to the extent she wanted and in consequence had to be convinced by the doctor so that he continued to orbit her, he was now suddenly a man to be contested for.

– *Because from what you say your husband has not made love to you for some years. Since it isn't from physical causes, it's obvious the man has found relief with somebody else. That's why he isn't grumbling any more. That's what it must be.*

– *Are you telling me I ought to start investigating in case there's something going on where he works?*

– *No, I'm just telling you that the person out there* (pointing to the door) *isn't a toy you have put on a shelf or in the cupboard and you need not bother with any more. He must have his own needs and it's reasonable that he will be looking to. You must know that nobody is to be taken for granted. That is besides what kills a marriage dead: the attitude of taking the other for granted.*

It was now time to push the knife in deeper. To show her the value the other person may have that we gradually lose sight of:

– *But, there exist as we said, always the solution of divorce. Take your children and leave home.*

— *And where pray should I go? We made that home for us and the children. If he wants to live his life as you insist he does, let him get up and leave.*

— *In a divorce, property is usually divided up* (I said, gritting my teeth.)

— *He's probably made sure everything is in his name but I shall be bringing up his children and I have my rights. He can't throw me out into the street.*

— *Naturally he'll give you alimony for the next ten years until the children are of age. Then you'll be free to do whatever you like.*

— *What on earth are you saying, Doctor? What sort of scenario is that?*

— *Oh, I see. He will have his freedom as of now. But so can you. Do you work?*

— *No, I look after the home and the children… That's a lot of work. Besides, when we got married my husband told me he didn't want me to work anymore and to devote myself to him and the children we would have.*

— *What job did you have then?*

— *I was the secretary of a client of his. That's how we met.*

— *I would think when he proposed, you were happy about it.* (I was sounding condescending. I must automatically be feeling scorn for her in my mind. I had to pull myself together right away.)

— *Yes I was. I remember I was boasting to my girlfriends, and they were envious.*

— *It's a good thing they can't see you now! They would be sorry for you.*

— *No, I haven't let anything show. Everyone still thinks we have the best marriage. They still think I'm so lucky.*

— *You could be… It's up to you to make this marriage work again. If we neglect a relationship and don't foster it, it tends to die. The roads of married couples get to diverge whereas at some time they were parallel, going side by side. There is you see a world–wide law, of 'divergence' that splits couples apart.*

I parted my hands to show what I meant.

— *…if you don't want to allow your relationship to get stale because of the great sentimental gap, you have to make an active energetic effort to get back on track. From saying a genuinely warm "Good morning!" to bringing some flowers, some unexpected present, you may find it ridiculous and trite, but a relationship can be kept alive only with some effort expended. If it's left on automatic pilot, it is fated to be worn out and gradually to die out.*

— *Do you mean to say that not only should I not accuse him of being so indifferent to me, but that on top of it, I should cherish him!*

— *Yes I do. Because if you don't, someone else will.*

— *How you carry on about 'the other'!*

— *I'm saying it because your attitude shows me you don't really want to divorce him. Therefore your sole alternative is to get close to him again. If you do that, you'll realise that he will come close too. Everything in a relationship is reciprocal. If a move to closeness is made by one side, sooner or later there will be a response from the other.*

— *There are none so deaf, as those who will not hear.*

— *And one more thing: the move has to be made without expecting an immediate response. If it is done solely to test the other's responsiveness it will come to nothing. If I do something for the sole purpose of being valued by someone, it will very probably meet with indifference, especially when one's motives are suspected by the other. In your case, I think you should make repeated moves of coming close, without expecting anything in return. I'm certain that in a short while, you'll be surprised by how your husband's attitude will change. What you offer will be returned and in fact most often it is returned multiplied.*

My first message had been transmitted. She was an intelligent woman and she had got it. She understood she could not have it all her way. She too had to make an effort before it was too late. I then spoke to the husband about the efforts they should all make to save their marriage without, of course, targeting him or reproaching him. It seemed to shake him up a bit, because he was evidently resigned to the way things were and had never thought of divorcing.

Tact and diplomacy is needed, so as to show that in general lines I am on the side of the wife, while on the other hand not putting the blame on the husband. I have to weigh everything I say, carefully. My role is to offer alternative scenarios, of which either they have not thought or dare not think, where they might lead the persons. I merely hint at some scenarios and others I take to their ultimate limit. It is always so as to give them a fright and give an impetus to self–protective reactions.

Some people see things very superficially and easily threaten a separation, whereas others see a divorce as something quite out of reach and inconceivable. In the first case I point out that things are not easy out there, away from the security of marriage, whereas in the second I show them that they have an option: it is possible to have a happy life after a divorce.

So, after being 'aggressive' to the lady of this story, by painting the repercussions she would have from quitting the relationship and her marriage in lurid colours, I now showed her a luminous window. I presented an alternative scenario, of preservation of her marriage. Something other than what she had imagined, i.e. a story of continuing clashes and continuing complaints.

The tactics of Provocative Psychotherapy is constant thumping, but with calculated blows, successively on the nail and on the anvil. The object is to bring out the contrasts and the extreme scenarios, so that the person treated should choose the least painful in the given circumstances.

In the process, the doctor has the opportunity to ascertain the true intentions, as well as the abilities of the patient. By describing the extreme scenarios at their limits, one can see how they react and if a person is able to take one or the other road. If one course scares them away, of their own initiative, they will opt for the other alternative.

Disorientation and relaxation

HOWEVER, it is not a good idea to grab a patient by the throat from the beginning, that is, to be aggressive from the start so that, although they expect their visit to the psychiatrist to be an occasion to tell their troubles and be justified, they are faced instead with provocation and aggression, from the outset.

What I usually do, is that when they start telling me their story I find an opportunity to draw their attention away from what they came to say. If for instance they tell me about where they grew up or the work they do or did, to ask for details:

– *What a nice town Kavala is. I was there recently and was impressed…*

– *Thessaloniki is the place to experience the student life. They are a large community and… all of them away from the family…*

– *A chef? How come you aren't fat? How do you manage, to be into food and not taste it all the time…*

– *Dressmaker? You must have made a name for yourself…*

In that way, I draw the patient's attention away from what is on their mind, which as is to be expected is stressful, not only to harmless subjects but especially to subjects I suspect are pleasant. This not only relaxes a patient who is seeing the psychiatrist for the first time, it also prepares the ground for the therapeutic alliance that is required in every medical situation.

The doctor's interest must of course be genuine, not fake and superficial, because it will be seen straight away by the patient, who may feel offended. Then, instead of good relations it may cause a gap and permanent rift between the doctor and the patient.

And why should the interest be really genuine? By means of this painless and distracting chatting I have learnt things that amazingly enriched my encyclopaedic knowledge. And at first hand, what's more: From cookery recipes to techniques for fishing and astrological analysis, interesting knowledge that at the same time relaxes and wins over the patient who has the feeling of chatting with a friend.

The approval

I HAVE at times realised that while the person sitting opposite me has in many ways expressed their detestation of their way of life, they nevertheless dare not change it. Timidity and fear of the unknown keeps many people imprisoned on courses that they not only dislike, but also do not deserve.

In such instances a 'shove' is needed for someone to take the heroic decision to change. In such cases I think that in the end the therapist's neutrality is detrimental to the person treated. Very often someone who comes to a psychiatrist is basically seeking an excuse to make a move. If I judge that such a move really is for the good of their mental economy and will not have them fall apart mentally, but will be of practical assistance, e.g. financially, then not only do I give them their excuse, I also give my encouraging approval.

I believe this is the doctor's role. He or she is the specialist who does not only have the knowledge – but also the necessary distance – so as to be able to form the optimum opinion. That, I stress again, is of course as long as complete neutrality is ensured. No emotionally involvement with the patient's state. This means the doctor has to be able to distinguish the solutions chosen for him or herself, from the solution best suited to the person asking for help.

Although it should go without saying, it is very often unfortunately not applied. For example a doctor who does not have the courage to leave a relationship, will dissuade anyone else asking for their help from separation and divorce. At the other extreme are divorced colleagues, who advise all their patients without exception to divorce too, irrespective of whether they are in a psychological – or even social and financial – condition to be able to.

Advice given with prudence, however, or rather, the approval given to what is the apparent desire of the patient – what he basically wishes – is in my opinion the duty of the doctor. This is besides what the patient has come to us for. That is why they pay us: to have the counsel of the specialist.

You cannot imagine the importance of the role of the approval of a person esteemed, as is the case of the doctor for the patient. It is worth adding a parenthesis on this particular aspect:

When I was practicing Consultation Psychiatry in a general hospital, that is examining and treating the mental state of patients hospitalised there, my colleagues asked me to examine a girl who was hospitalised with atypical symptoms of abdominal discomfort. She was a courteous person whose eyes showed desolation. Her look was glum and melancholy. Although she was in bed, one could see she was strong with a well exercised body structure. This showed more when I fetched a chair and sat next to her bed, which made her sit up and rest her back against the bedstead. I noticed then not only how mobile she was but also certain masculinity in her movements.

Although she was unwilling to talk to me, I got her to overcome her hesitation and open up to me. When they hear the word 'psychiatrist', many patients button up. They become guarded and answer questions in monosyllables. Some even become paranoid: "Who sent you and why? Do they think I'm insane?"

Here I follow the strategy of beginning from easy subjects, purely medical: "Why are you in hospital? When did the pain start? Where is it exactly? How long does it last?" Focusing on purely physical symptoms places the doctor in a medical frame and cancels the perception – which prevails unfortunately – that the psychiatrist is something else. For most people psychiatry is closer to Philosophy, Theology and Metaphysics than Medicine. This is also what makes people generally wary. I sometimes realise it is easier for a doctor to say to a patient that they should be seen by an oncologist than a psychiatrist!

The next step of approach is to investigate the timing of the connection of the physical symptoms to some mental trauma occurring in the patient's life. In fact, to muddy the water even more, first I ask if the symptoms began at a time of physical tiredness. The standard answer from all the patients is that at the time when the physical trouble started they were not only under physical but mental strain too. Furthermore, the patient needs to talk about the problem. They just do not want to be labelled crazy, that their symptoms are in their mind alone, that they want to be pitied or 'get their way'.

So, when I asked this girl with the masculine movements what had caused physical or mental tiredness six months ago when the bodily trouble began, she looked at me for a while with an exploratory gaze, as if she were weighing whether she could confide her secret to me. After what seemed to me a long pause, she took a deep breath and started telling me her story, which she had perhaps never told anybody else before.

She had grown up and lived in a large provincial town near Athens. Her father was a solicitor, comfortably off, with a status of prestige in the small community of that town. She is an only child and was brought up with strict rules of morality. As soon as she began puberty and to have a bosom and curves, her parents would did not allow her to go around with boys. She could not go to a coffee shop, cinemas or dances and parties without her mother. For her, the transformation into womanhood seemed as something terrible that practically put her in prison. In her family the image of a woman was something vulgar, sordid and to be scorned.

In order to escape from that prison the girl refused anything female about herself and gradually acquired a rather masculine behaviour. She played tennis and worked out intensively, getting a strapping muscular figure. At the same time she developed a close friendship with another girl a little younger. Since she could not go out with boys she shared the tenderness and care that was innate in her with this girlfriend.

— *Of course because of the explosion of hormones that happens in puberty…*

That was my first comment, interrupting the flow of her account. I gave her a medical excuse for what was obviously bothering her. Then I went on immediately, trying to facilitate her confession now that I could tell what direction she was taking.

— *…it's quite natural that a sentimental relationship should develop between you.*

— *Neither of us realised what was happening. The two of us are so close…*

— *You could call it being in love.*

— *I dare not call it that. But we are something like sisters… Others see us as sisters, but for us it's something else.*

— *Well, you see, hormones have to burst out.*

I spoke in as natural a tone of voice as possible, levelly, without a trace of criticism or irony. I was expressionless, as if my face muscles were a mask, my body immobile, frozen, I didn't blink an eye. I think that is where the whole game was won. As was normal, she had been afraid of criticism, but not only did I not pass a negative judgment, I gave her biological explanations for her great secret problem. So she opened up to me.

— *We both of us had… an orgasm together for the first time. We have become one. We breathe together…*

— *What about your parents?*

— *That's exactly the problem now. For the past year they've been constantly pressing me to get married. I'm past thirty and they insist, they point to various men of our acquaintances. They haven't understood anything about me. It's a well-kept secret, that because of their insistence I shall have to reveal to them.*

— *So what? What can happen? At first they'll be astounded, but then they'll have to take you as you are, or rather how they forced you to become…*

Suddenly, she beamed. It was like a rainbow after rain. She gave me a broad smile. It was the best gift of the day for me. One more satisfied client, I thought, mocking myself. You see, I am always having dialogues with my inner self, satirising what I see, what I say and what I think.

– *I hadn't thought of it that way. It was a rope choking me. I kept seeing an impasse closing in on me. There was nothing but a wall in front of me… Now I can see that there is life behind the wall after all.*

– *And in any case, Athens is close by. Who obliges you to live in your town? You can live in Athens the way you want to, with whomever you like and visit your parents as often as you wish.*

– *Doctor, thank you so much. You have taken such a weight off my mind…*

Two days later the patient left the hospital. I would not have known the outcome of my intervention, had I not seen her by chance three years later in the corridor of the same hospital. She recognised me and came to say hello.

– *I'll never forget what you said. I had never imagined I could reveal such things and not be scolded. Until that day when I talked to you, I used to feel guilty towards everyone. After what you said, not only did I tell my parents, we didn't even have to leave town. My friend and I live there and are accepted by the society… Anyway, we think so.*

She laughed, and I went away smiling with satisfaction, trying as always to hide my feelings. From that moment on, however, I realised that I could say something that would bring about a major change in a person's life. Many people go through life vacillating, between decisions they do not have the courage to make. They waste years being tormented on the horns of a dilemma. Dilemmas they often cannot so much as formulate.

A psychiatrist has the duty to help people pinpoint them. And, of course to take the decisions that suit them best.

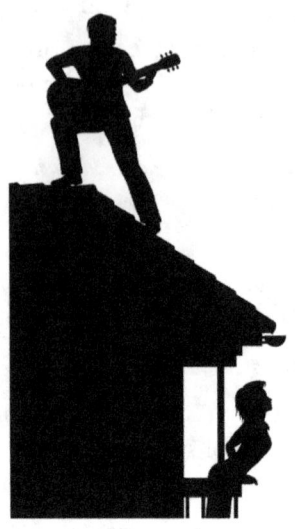

RELATIONS BETWEEN THE TWO SEXES

ONE DAY my friend Mary told me about a surprise party her boyfriend John had organised. He wanted them to get married for some time now. The party was for her birthday, and when she came home and opened the door she found about twenty friends of hers whom John had invited. He had seen to everything, organising the catering with food, drink, waiters and a DJ. He had even told the friends to park some way away from her address so that Mary would not guess anything, when she came home. As she told me about it, she was not only delighted, she was touched too.

I have to admit it, I was envious when I heard that. It is not something that is done every day, especially by men. As a gesture it shows great love or… a strong motivation. It was this last that gave my heart a pinch. I didn't say anything about this to my friend who had come to see me a couple of times because, in the past year she had been irritable and was slightly depressed. She was already 39 years old and was not married, nor of course did she have a child. She had been absorbed in her job and the family business and was also rather reticent whenever an approach was made to her, because her family name was well known and she was very wealthy. Although she was sociable she did not open up easily, being afraid, and not without reason, that whoever approached her, had some financial objective in mind.

For the last month, she told me, John had been sleeping with her in Mary's comfortable flat in a smart quarter of Athens. He was well off, but his finances were far from being comparable to Mary's fortune. At the time, John was an executive in a big firm and his acquaintance and later his relationship with Mary were admittedly a great opportunity for him.

That surprise party had been the catalyst for Mary's defences to fall. My friend bloomed, got married a few months later, and had a baby the next year already. John quit his job and joined Mary's family's business, in essence taking Mary's place in her professional duties.

However, he made the mistake so many people make: he felt he had security and thought he was 'sitting pretty'. He gradually neglected his wife and though he did not realise it, in himself he was gradually demeaning her. When he met her, she was a dynamic businesswoman and she now appeared as merely an ordinary housewife and mother.

I heard that John's father-in-law later died and John was running the business. I did not hear anything about them for years. I saw Mary once at a social gathering and almost did not recognise her. She had got fat, and as I noticed, was drinking too much.

Until the day, about ten years later, when I heard John's voice over the phone. He wanted an urgent meeting to discuss something personal. He came to my office that same afternoon. He was agitated and seemed desperate. He told me his relationship with his wife had been in crisis for the last years. Mary had become hard and was looking for opportunities to pick a fight. In fact they had recently been fighting all the time. Mary does not even respect the child's presence and has often told John to leave the home. The day before, she had instructed the household help to pack up John's belongings and throw him out of the house. He spent the night at his mother's and had come today to ask my advice.

He was in panic and in despair.

– *You have to do something. Mary is not herself. She's destroying our life. Our family… the way she's going she'll break everything up.*

– *But you're o.k., thank God. You're well and strong and your life can go on without her. Also your daughter is a big girl now and I don't think she'll have a problem if her parents separate.*

– *What are you saying? I came to you to tell me how to get her back… can't you see I need her… I can't live without her any more.*

– *Why can't you live without Mary? Are you telling me you're good for nothing and that it's Mary who supports you?*

— No, I'm not saying that. But she's become indispensable to me.

— In what way? For sex?

— That has been eliminated from our life. We haven't had sex in about three years now.

— What? And how do you deal with that?

— It just happened... Both of us gave up on it... Well, you might as well know, during the time I did have some transient sexual relations.

— So what's the point of keeping this marriage, which it seems to me, is only a prison for you? You're living with a woman who doesn't want you and on top of it, you think she's crazy. You have quarrels and clashes every day over big or little issues. And what's more, you have no sexual relations. I think Mary has given you the best chance to escape from your prison.

— And how am I to manage, on my own?

— If you mean financially, I don't think you'll have any difficulty finding a job. You might not earn as much as you are today from Mary's businesses, but you're very capable and you have a good reputation in the market as a successful manager.

— Yeah, I hear you. D'you think I haven't thought of that too? But to be honest, no job can give me the sort of lifestyle I have now.

— If by lifestyle you mean holidays, travel, smart restaurants and receptions, then yes. But on the other hand you'll have your freedom. You won't have Mary getting on your nerves, as you say she is and you'll be able to have any girlfriend you like. Just don't forget that freedom has a price. It's never given for free. There's always something in exchange for liberation. Many gave their blood fighting for freedom. Liberty demands sacrifices. And you don't have to make a lot. Yes, I understand you'll be less comfortable. But think what you'll gain. Look ahead. As if the company you worked for, closed down and you have other opportunities in front of you. New perspectives. A future that could be worse, but could also be better. You're facing a new challenge. Look at it positively and you won't lose. You have all the capacities.

— I have to say I'm feeling a little more optimistic.

It seems our talk really did help him. From feeling totally dependent on Mary and Mary's business, he dared to see alternative ways out and that he could stand on his own feet. Although he paid a reasonable price, because as he confesses much later, he had been very impressed by what I had said about 'liberty having a price'.

This boost to his self–confidence, apparently also had an effect on Mary's perception of him. Her stance toward John changed. Just as, when someone takes something you may have thrown out, that thing suddenly acquires value, in the same way Mary began seeing him in a different perspective. It was she, who had rejected him and in fact the more he demonstrated his dependence on her, the more she rejected him. When however she saw, he could stand alone and could very well leave her, John suddenly acquired value for her. So she evidently simmered down. Not only did she 'tolerate' him, she tried to be more attractive. She went on a diet and exercised and became once more the Mary I used to know.

This is how John kept his relationship: when he felt strong and was ready to quit it. This is in no way a paradox. The story of this relationship is unfortunately not unusual. On the contrary, it's extremely commonplace. One may even say the way this turned out is the rule for human relationships.

In societies where the choice of a companion is free, people struggle to find the best possible one. The 'best' corresponds to the criteria we have in mind which, of course, have been formed in us by our family and social environment. When we have succeeded in catching the best possible mate, it is the rule that we then feel we have conquered, and relax our effort to attract our companion.

Women, who although before marriage are careful of their appearance every time they are meeting their future husband, often change after marriage. They progressively neglect themselves. They go round the house without doing their hair and look a mess. Although before marriage, when they were with their mate they wore provocative clothes and underwear, afterwards they wear a carelessly buttoned dressing–gown and worn slippers. It's no exaggeration. It is sadly the rule. Marriage transforms a woman into someone 'yoked'. Often after the first child is born a lot of them not only feel they are now secure but, as a friend of mine with experience of such things says, that they 'have made sure of their social security'.

Of course, the equivalent happens with men too. They get flabby, they do not watch their manners, pick their ears and noses, belch and walk around in worn pyjamas. It is to be expected, that as time goes on they will forget anniversaries and birthdays and forget to buy presents and give their 'once' beloved a surprise.

The truth is that when a couple feels they are two animals under the same yoke, they stop courtship. They just try to pull the cart called family. As a matter of fact in time all they care about is how to exert the least effort. So they often compete as to who has the right to contribute the least to the daily family chores.

This day–to–day bargaining is detrimental to a relationship. It is clearly better for chores to be shared out from the start; who will load the washing machine and who will take the rubbish out. Negotiation leads to clashes and those in turn to cracks in the bonds that keep the couple united.

All the entire above scene is a result of the social relations connected with marriage. In Western societies until recently a marriage was a tie broken only with difficulty. It was a stable contract, that always had some clauses of course, but they were in tiny letters to be called on only in exceptional circumstances.

Divorce was rare fifty years ago. Married couples maintained their yoke for better or worse.

It has to be said that this brought a security which, however, carried an abdication from the other's demands. As the values of the two companions are usually different, the relations are then one–sided. As time passes one of the two seems better–looking, or more intelligent or wealthier than the other. Consequently, unavoidably the bonds of marriage become the bonds of dependency. One feels dependent on the other. Not that that is a bad thing. What is bad is, when one realises the other is entirely dependent on them and hanging round their neck. Then not only do they feel the other is a burden but, they will soon demystify the other and demean them. Unfortunately, from initially admiring one's companion, one gradually comes to tolerate them.

There is only one way to avoid this ineluctable development. Accepting that at any moment the other is free to go. Since frequently marriage turns into a golden cage or is merely convenient – whether psychologically or financially – only preparedness for freedom to be claimed can avert the destructive wear and tear of the relationship.

In the example of Mary and John, only when the dependent member, John, showed he could stand alone, claiming his freedom, then and only then, did Mary begin taking account of him and claiming him. It is no coincidence that so many love songs of the world have the words 'you left' or 'why did you leave me' and suchlike. I for one do not know any that says "… while you were with me, I didn't pay attention to you". But unfortunately experience teaches that it is the most frequent reason for 'leaving'.

Cohabitation is like labour relations; when there is permanency, productivity falls precipitately. There is a term in Greek for 'typically civil–servant'. It is scornful, describing the total absence of initiative to be productive of civil servants who consider their job and their salary as a sine qua non, with the cover of permanency given to civil servants. In the same way, when one of a married couple considers it a given, if not actually mandatory, that the other will keep their part in the marriage regardless of anything, they lose every motive to attract them, thus let go of themselves and lose their attractiveness.

True, as in labour relations, the retort to the 'civil servant' mentality is that absence of permanency often brings insecurity. But, just as the economy through its history answered this dilemma definitively, so does society give an answer making the bonds of wedlock ever more fragile. As time goes by, human relations are less a given and less permanent.

This is not necessarily a bad thing. On the contrary, it obliges relationships to preserve their dynamism. This is certainly more arduous but, unfortunately all good things have a cost. For a relationship to stay a good one and above all alive, an effort is required. Both have to exert energy. Not obligatorily in the same amount, but from both sides. They should both of them try, with words and acts – that maybe do not come easily – to keep the warmth of their relationship. Before, and mainly after, marriage. And they should know that if they relax their efforts, they will pay a much higher price than their temporary gain.

When biology is disregarded

SOME DAYS ago I went to a good restaurant with my wife. I sat down at the table the maitre d' showed us to and, curious animal that I am, cast an exploratory look around. A party of three women aged about thirty was sitting next to us. Further away at another table there were five young women and at another a group of four ladies about fifty years old. There were also two couples in the restaurant sitting together, and another couple on their own who left early , evidently so as to 'have a good time' as my wife observed.

In the past few years this is something one sees ever more often. Young women on their own, from age twenty upward and even over forty. Women: looking for the man of their life. Sadly, unsuccessfully, to the point where some of them give up in the end and abandon the effort. Or, on reaching 35, which for most women constitutes an age limit for child bearing, they make a major concession and marry the first guy who knocks at their door!

Some young women, pretty as a picture, come to my office, who are in despair because 'they can't find a good man'. It is evident that "something is rotten in the kingdom of Denmark". Relations between young people have been disjointed by the changes that have taken place in modern Western society. The entry of women into the job market that came about mainly after World War II, unavoidably entailed equality of the sexes: the same pay for the same work.

But competition in the work arena that also, unavoidably, intensified between men and women, altered the identity of both sexes. Women tend to put their femininity aside and act the 'tough guy', or else they exploit their feminine 'advantages', but in a cold and calculating way that unfortunately strips them of their physical authenticity.

Young women have ceased to be the enchanting beings that the princes of fairy tales strive to conquer. They have shed their attractiveness. In any case, attraction is a term interwoven with passivity. So from the moment when women became actors it followed that from being prey they should become hunters.

What I wish to clarify here is that what occurred in man's societies recently was not natural, that is, it was not according to the rules of nature. It merely satisfied the demands of the financial relations upon which the organised human societies were founded. I am saying that it is not a rule of nature that the male should hunt the female. In nature it is on the contrary: the male peacock is who spreads his tail so as to attract the female. In most animal species it is the males who sing or… bellow, for the females to hear and approach, at a time, of course, when they are in a period of fertility for breeding. The female then examines the male carefully and if he meets with her approval – always from the angle of eugenics – she will allow the male his erotic embraces.

It means that in nature, it is the female who is responsible for making a choice. The whole of evolution, through physical selection, depends of the choices of the females. They will choose the strongest, the tallest, the handsomest and, in our day, the most successful males. It was the female animals who, with their selectivity, guided the evolution of life on our planet from the amoeba to the human being. For millions of years the burden of development was borne by the females.

It is besides not by chance, that the early societies of humans were matriarchies. The mothers were the chiefs. They made love with whatever men they chose, and had children, who belonged to them. Men did not have children of their own. They were all something like uncles to the children. No man knew if a child was his. The hunter men cared for all the children and the women of the community. And hunting was in any case a group activity then.

This changed with the appearance of agriculture and later, animal husbandry. The man who cleared and cultivated a field, wanted to pass it on to his own descendants. Not to let the community have it. It was the fruit of his toil and it was natural that he should want to give it to his beloved family. In this way, the matriarchy broke up into small family units. The man farmer isolated a woman, with whom he had children. In fact, so to make absolutely sure that the children were his he tried to shut his wife away completely. He built his own private dwelling and in essence imprisoned his wife away from the rest of the community. The family agricultural business was born. All the children helped in the work of the field, cultivation, harvesting and processing of the produce. The field, and later the stable and the animals were in the possession of the family, which property had to be passed down to the heirs, as was the custom. The heirs therefore had to be truly of the same blood. Any doubt as to the blood relationship was a bomb at the foundations of the familial structure of society.

This regime has come down to our days. Property is inherited and consequently the blood line has to be pure and indisputable. For this the wife–mother has to be above all faithful. The divine Commandment 'Thou shalt not commit adultery' is precisely the result of this social structuration. Society is now male–dominated. The man has the possessions. It is therefore he, who has the power and from now on he, who makes the choice of a wife. In this way, the woman, who was the judge and the selector of men was turned into the prey of the man.

The alteration of the social role of the sexes obliged the woman to be attractive. What we call femininity today is not constitutional in the woman. It is the outcome of social relations of only the last few thousand years. At the same time it also demands the existence of freedom of the citizens: freedom of choice of one's companion.

We know that today still in many societies a woman does not have to be attractive and 'feminine'. Marriage, this social contract, takes place without the slightest participation of the woman. In some cases as a matter of fact it occurs without the participation of the husband in question even. The bride is chosen by the parents and the husband has never seen the bride. So the woman has no cause to be attractive and beautiful. That is of course another infringement of the law of natural selection and evolution. It is the way ill–favoured, inferior and deficient humans proliferate who, in natural selection would be outside of the selective process.

In the Western 'civilised' society the falsification of natural selection is to be found in the wallet the man carries. It is no secret that women look men first in their pocket and then in the eyes and the remaining ingredients of good looks. They do not really care if he is short or cannot run very fast or is not well–built. What they are more interested in is that he should be able to support her and the children she will have with him.

I am not criticising them for that. In a society in which financial insecurity is predominant on the one hand, as well as consumerism on the other, it follows that someone should place financial ease first. What use are the good looks of a husband who is not in a position to pull the family cart that the young woman envisions?

It could be said at this point that a rich man may have the brains and abilities indispensable for our society's upward mobility. Thus, in consequence, modern woman promotes the development of these qualities by her choices. However, albeit that could partially be valid for the self–made man, it certainly does not apply to those who inherited financial wealth who moreover constitute the majority of rich young men. In their case natural selection and evolution meet their downfall.

But when women entered into productivity, initially in the industrial society and later the post–industrial one and where the working woman's income has to a degree come to equal a man's, the equilibrium altered dramatically. In Western Europe and North America more and more women are now financially independent. This, as was to be expected, planted a bomb in the foundations of the institution of marriage, at least as it was known until now. There are nowadays not a few women who can financially support the only child that corresponds to them. In this of course a welfare state has greatly helped, that has been developed over the years. One result of this is the scary quantity of divorces. Nowadays, a financially independent woman is not prepared to put up with her husband's faults and thus easily maps out her own route.

As to the number of children a woman bears, that diminished, not only because she came into the work market but also, because of the lofty demands that our over–consumerist society makes. Children have needs: from expensive diapers to expensive schools and colleges.

Therefore, the bourgeois family cannot support a large number of children. Their number can in no way be compared to how many a farming society had, who besides helped in the family income.

In parallel, a further factor struck the fatal blow to the institution of the family: as we have seen, the patriarchal family was the result of possessions and the need to bequeath them. But in our day the increase of expectations from extended life has in essence done away with inheritance. Why should someone wait for the father to die, at 85, to inherit the family field or the house? Since, furthermore, the person in question will themselves be over 55 and it will follow that when they reach that age they will not only already have formed a family of their own, but will probably be oriented toward a pension. Nobody in our day in most Western countries where life expectation is over 75 can base their life plans on their right of inheritance to the paternal fortune.

Although I am sorry to say it, I have come across several cases of the offspring of rich families who made the mistake of basing their life's programme on the family inheritance alone, or young people with wealthy aunts without issue waiting for them to die so as to enjoy their inheritance. What happened that God gave the elderly relatives generous numbers of years of life, in the course of which, what is more, they became ever more careful not to let go of a penny of their fortune because of the insecurity that grows with age. And not a few of them, who were wealthy, took care in their later life to spend their assets so as to have the best life they could! They are in no way to be reproached, who have every right to enjoy every penny they earned by their hard work. Reproach is due to those, who waited mouth wide open, beneath the family tree for the 'ripe fruit' of their inheritance to fall.

I have personal knowledge of an instance when two bridegrooms who had married a handsomely financially endowed bride died successively one after the other. The bride–daughter, twice widowed, is 80 today and her wealthy father is 105 (!) keeping a tight hold of the reins of his enormous fortune. The daughter, who after all this broke off relations with her over–centenarian father, tries to stand on her own feet and support herself, while her papa is cared for by young and well paid maids!

It is clear that as much as the expectations for an extended life are on the rise, the dependence on inheritance declines correspondingly. Therefore, so does the necessity for ensuring paternity, the fundamental element of the patriarchal family as it was: simply, it loses its importance. Nowadays, we are rapidly approaching the preponderance of the single parent family. In most cases it is in the form of the mother and her one or two children. The mother brings up these children with the assistance on the one hand of the social structures offered by modern society and on the other of various companions or a husbands that she selects, however with no long–term and exclusive commitment. Furthermore this last is no longer necessary to the degree that it was in the classic patriarchal family.

Consequently, as modern young women work at this scenario, what they take greater care of is their career. This is what will make them strong and independent in their future life: Strong enough to support their children, even without the help of a man. Above all though, they feel independent of any male repression and control on their life.

However, another side to this scenario to be expected is that child–bearing will come later. Most young women today go to college, enter the professional arena and compete with men on equal terms. This naturally obliges them to put off marriage and especially having children. Also, since in the past few years, progress in medicine through in vitro insemination, has extended the child–bearing age, women in their thirties are less worried that the end of their fertility is knocking at their door.

Not that a change has taken place in nature. It is well known that in the human species the capacity of a female to be pregnant and complete her pregnancy successfully diminishes after the age of 18 – 20. After the age of 30, this capacity diminishes by geometric progression. This is why in our society young women are led to situations with no way out. They have closed their ears to the tolling of the biological bell of child–bearing and multiplication of the species.

Moreover, something that has further contributed to this is what we call the 'sexual revolution'. After the contraceptive pill was produced in the 60s the act of sex has been entirely disconnected from childbearing. Sexual pleasure has become an independent objective, irrespective of the motive of fertility. The value of sexual satisfaction has been inflated and in modern society has become an objective on its own.

The interest of young people is focused on obtaining their sexual satisfaction alone and not on completing the process of fertility. The latter has become a synonym of bonds and obligations, understandably contrary to the ideal of freedom and independence which is what young men and women look for after the age of 16. Indeed, in our day, young people do not want obligations, they want to enjoy love–making without the burdens of a family.

Unfortunately, in a post–industrial society young women let themselves be aware of the ringing of the bell of fertility only after the mid–thirties. Until then their attention is directed to having a good time and acquiring independence through financial ease. Innumerable are the times I have heard them say: "I'm not going to let getting married interfere with making a success of my life" when I ask them why they don't marry, meaning they will not abandon or interrupt their career, which is like a hunt, and is in a critical phase, to hunt for a husband!

Nevertheless, a woman's biological clock never stops ticking and does not wait for the proper social and financial circumstances to be in good order.

Fortunately for a man the situation is different. Biology behaves with more gallantry to him. As the male stud, he can do the job nature has assigned to him well after the age of forty. The quality of sperm may diminish slightly with age, but a man does not face the stigma of being unable to produce offspring. Indeed, with the discovery on the one hand of medicine that enhances erection and on the other the prolongation of life expectancy, in our day men can produce children even when they are far over 40. They function as lovers well into old age and they can still live to see their children grow, marry and give them grandchildren if they get to the seventh or even eighth decade.

The outcome of all these essential social changes is that women aged 25 to 35 do not find the mates corresponding to their expectations, because, obviously, at that age men have not yet matured professionally. Unfortunately, most young men are unable to support a family, in the style demanded by young women of the modern bourgeois class.

Therefore, the selection made by these women turns to older men. But on the other hand, when a man reaches a level in his career, when after all he can satisfy the increased demands of such women, understandably his interest is directed to much younger women, not only because of the fresher appearance of a 25–year old than when she is 35, but also because of her better capacity for child–bearing.

This considerable difference between the sexes, which with time increases, has brought about new conditions in their relationships. When a young woman belatedly seeks a mate–husband with whom to have a baby, she already has a sufficient experience of life. She has usually been to college, has met a number of men and acquired financial assets. Also, after having studied and survived in the professional world, she is familiar with competing with the opposite sex.

She has developed judgment. She will not easily buy the line that every man tries to sell her. This may seem to be a sensible attitude, since she is not easily fooled, nor impressed. But on the other hand, it does lead to demystification of the opposite sex and this brings her alas to an inner solitude. There are not enough men to play the fairy tale prince with which all little girls grew up. The modern thirty–something–year–old woman, and it is a pity, can see that 'the king is naked'.

I say it is a pity because falling in love is based on fairy tales. On what we believe about the other, not what they really are. This is why the passion of love does not last. We ourselves often make up an image of the other, in accordance with our own desires and aspirations. And what else is 'love at first sight' but an ephemeral impression we receive, according to what we wish to see in the other?

This is the reason why passionate love very rarely lasts long: because as time goes by, being close and in contact, we realise what is going on behind the façade, behind the scene. We see the other's true dimension and not what we had attributed to them. Therefore, for the passion to be sustained both have to cherish the myth that one 'sold' to the other, at the beginning of the relationship.

Here I remember something personal to me: a talk I had with my daughter some years ago. She was complaining that she could not find a boyfriend with whom she 'clicked', as she put it.

– *I wonder what he has to have to impress you, I said to her. Can't you see you have castrated the boys? When you leave a nightclub and the young man you met offers to drive you home and you say 'no thanks, I have my own car', what do you expect him to do? What's more, when he sees you getting into the two–seater sports car you ask me to buy for you he won't come near you again. That's the reason I told you to get a little city car. I'm telling you again, ask them sometimes to come and fetch you from home in their car. Don't show right away that you're independent.*

– *But what if I am?*

– *Think that a relationship is a game, a theatrical game. Be the stage director. Let the other play the role which actually is what you want from him. Get in the car and let him drive. Be relaxed in the co–driver's seat and show him some confidence. Try not to castrate him. Don't make criticisms of his driving. Let him feel a man, powerful and a leader. I'm not saying close your eyes. The art is being in control of everything, without it showing.*

– *You mean as in families of old, where although they were essentially matriarchal the women did not appear at all?*

– *Women have always been the boss of the family. Men merely brought home the cash and they went to war.*

– *But Daddy, nowadays the women also bring back the money. So they have the right to have more to say in the family.*

– *This is the mistake most people make. A family should not be a field of antagonism. The family should be seen as a team. If the players fight to keep the ball longest the team will lose. The ball must go to the one who at each stage is better equipped to help the most. A goal keeper does not shoot goals, but if his team wins, so does he. Don't forget that to share in a game is as meaningful as scoring.*

– *If that's so, we really are playing the game wrong. We try to keep the ball and score instead of giving it to the man for him to score.*

– *I don't know if it's unfortunate for you, but you now have become very capable at scoring. However, on the other hand the boys have grown up with the myth that it is they who score and that their masculinity is judged by it. So, if they don't score, they feel impotent. You and your girlfriends take the ball and then… you expect the boys to hit on you. Big mistake. And then we are surprised by some girls from an impoverished background who steal your boyfriends. That's just because they give them the ball and cheer him when he scores. That's what a man wants. They make a man feel powerful, while you make them feel impotent.*

– *But then Dad, why did you urge me to study and acquire so many advantages?*

– *For you to have self–esteem. But although you must appreciate your strength, you must keep it under control. You don't have to show your worth all the time. That you have to is neither your fault nor mine. Our society has changed. You women have come up in the world and that scares us. When I was a student and went out with your mother for the first time, I was driving the family car. Your mother, who was also a student, was impressed because they didn't have a car in her family. Just as she was impressed when we went to Rome and to Paris the first time and I was showing her the cities I knew thanks to my parents. And now, you my daughter have your own car and we have been to most of the major cities of Europe and North America. I wonder, what does a young man have to do to impress you?*

– *What are you trying to tell me? That it's wrong to have an education and experiences?*

– *No, I'm not, but for girls of your social class to be impressed and live the myth, they must either be taken out in sports cars and taken up and down in private jets and helicopters, or put on a motorbike and whizzed off to pretentious and extreme situations. But both extremes are usually disastrous:*

In the first case it's a game for rich spoiled brats from wealthy families, a state of excess and decadence, where everything has already been tried and, often, is combined with drugs. I want you to keep one thing in mind: that there's no such thing as money that never come to an end. As you know, there are lots of rich families who made mistakes and ended up not being able to buy food.

In the other case, the players are young 'boheme' fellows who are marginal. That's why girls from bourgeois backgrounds are impressed unconventional types whom your mother would call good–for–nothing or terrorists, or 'artists' in the bad sense– guys who can't earn their living and therefore are looking for living as a parasite on some woman.

I have often had to tell young girls these preoccupations of mine when they asked for my help because they felt they were in an impasse. It is true that nowadays in the relations between the sexes things are much more complicated than they were a generation or two ago. We are in a phase of transition. Society is changing and the challenges as well as the dead ends are increased. It is necessary to understand the changes in social roles and similar manoeuvres. One cannot proceed in the new conditions with the old, tried and tested models. We have to make new ones and experiment on these.

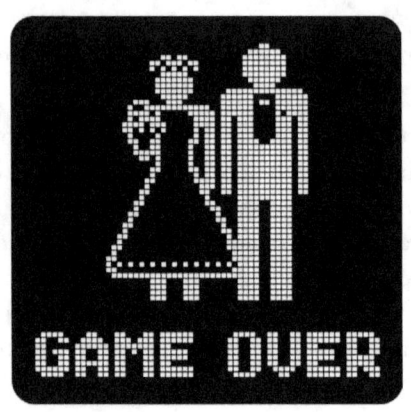

DIVORCE: A WAR FOR FREEDOM

AN ACQUAINTANCE of my wife's, Zoe, rang me up. She wanted to see me about a serious personal matter. I had met Zoe in Courchevel in France, where I went skiing in the Christmas holidays. She was a slim, pretty woman aged about 40, married to a decent and pleasant man, Alex, who said he was 65. He dyed his hair and tried to follow us on skis, but… age will tell. He wanted to go to bed early at night, but most annoying was that he had to have lunch at a certain time and then have a siesta. We would be having a good run and were warmed up when the couple would leave us to go back to the hotel.

Obviously, my wife and I commented on this. A first we said it must be an excuse to go to their room to make love. Of course we were remembering our youth when we looked for pretexts to be alone together. We saw the most optimistic aspect and were perhaps envious.

But a couple of days later Zoe told Alex to go back to the hotel alone. I realised then that she had engineered it so that at that moment we were on a ski run that passed in front of the hotel so that it should seem natural for him to go back alone. She stayed with us and we continued skiing, almost until the lifts stopped. Zoe was a proficient skier and seemed happy to be with us. My wife and I looked at one another and concluded in common, without saying much, that the woman was trapped. "This is what happens to those who get involved with older men!" was the philosophical dictum of us both. I did not miss the opportunity to remind my wife that her own first husband had been a lot older than she was.

I'm sorry to say that my job makes me abrupt sometimes at the wrong moment. My manner of approach to my patients, when I want them to see their own failings, in a rather brutal way so as to provoke their reaction with the object of having them improve, has unfortunately infiltrated into my personal life. I realise, although most times too late, that I have been nasty and have hurt people I love. Hurt friends or even social acquaintances, who have after all not asked for my help to change their ways. So I have no reason to be abrupt with them. Regrettably, my behaviour only provokes in them a reflex of defensive distancing.

However, although I am aware of it, nevertheless my profession has influenced me so much that I cannot refrain from my sharp comments. As a dentist will look at everyone's teeth, so do I, unwittingly, explore the other's character, bringing out their weak points that in my opinion need improvement. And sadly, at times words escape me when they should not.

So, when Zoe came to my office, she confided that she and her husband were not getting on at all well. She had married him when she was 28 and he 48. She was his secretary and at that time he was separating from his first wife. Alex was just starting out in business after leaving his father–in–law's, who was a ship–owner. In the early years Zoe was happy but she realised in time that what Alex gave her was perhaps security but not the tenderness and companionship she wanted. Alex was successful in business and provided a life of exceptional financial comfort, but…

– I always had the feeling he was using me. From the moment we were having sex to when we went out. I felt he was just showing me off to his friends, as a hunter displays the head of the tiger he shot. I was just an object for him. He was more occupied with his shops, even, because he worried that something could go wrong. So he took special care of them, while I was taken for granted: he took no notice of me. To buy a handbag I had to ask him again and again, and beg him. It has happened, I confess that I asked while we were having sex.

– Oh, why is that? Wasn't the sex in itself enough for you?

I asked in all innocence, as if I did not understand. Out of my professional perversion I hit people where it hurts, for them to break out of their limitations.

– Sex interests him only for his own satisfaction. In and out in two minutes and then he turns onto his other side. He doesn't care if I have any pleasure too. I told you, he just uses me. So some years now I don't want him to touch me. I sleep on the far edge of the bed, to be as far away from him as possible. I see him as a piece of meat lying beside me.

— *So why have you stayed with him for so long?*

— *Because I have to tell you I'm all alone ... and I haven't got a penny.*

There was silence for a moment. Her eyes began to fill with tears. I softened. I gave her a paper handkerchief and looked at her with sympathy and understanding. I said nothing and waited for Zoe to break her silence.

— *I haven't told you the worst. What really finished him as far as I was concerned: while I was expecting our daughter, George made a pass at my sister...*

— *Is she older or younger than you?*

I said this with professional detachment, in an indifferent way so as to lighten the atmosphere and to show that it was a commonplace for me. So my interlocutors often reveal a little bit of what is on their mind that they were concealing. If on the contrary I am too eager, they may take fright and retract the revelation they were about to make. If however I do not show emotion, or better, surprise, they proceed confidently to tell what is tormenting them.

In certain other cases they want to make an impression or to justify their stance which I have usually been criticising. So they try to find an important secret or some special piece of information, thinking it is the ace up their sleeve. When they throw it into the discussion they think they have won the game. After that, I shall justify them for not having the guts to separate, for instance, or have a life independent of their parents...

— *My sister is three years older and I'm afraid she too was 'coming on' to George. I haven't spoken to her since. I don't think they had a sexual relationship but the way my sister told me about it was like saying "it won't be my fault if I do something with your husband. He's the one making a pass." Don't you see? Instead of putting him in his place from the start, she was flattered to say the least... and allowed him to believe he could play around...*

— *Don't you have any other siblings?*

— *No brothers or sisters or father. My mother lives in the provinces and won't stand by me. She's sulking because I don't speak to my sister. She wants us to be loving or else 'she doesn't want to see me'. Nor will she accept the accusation against her eldest... I'm all alone.*

— *Yet despite all this you want to start a war?*

— *It's not war I want. It's my freedom.*

— *But freedom is not given away. It is conquered. And the struggle for freedom is never easy.*

— *I know. I'll lose the yacht in the summer and the luxury hotels. But I'll be able to sleep in a bed alone.*

— *It isn't that simple. I have heard about many divorces. None of them was a rose garden.*

Don't believe there is such a thing. Divorce is a war. You have to be well prepared so as not to lose it.

— I'll take the child with me and will have alimony for her, and I think he will give me alimony too, that I'll manage to have an amount of money.

— *Again it's not that simple'. The first thing that will happen — and you will remember this — is that he will claim the child.*

— Yes, that's right. When we talked about it first he said he would take on the child because he can afford to bring her up better. But for me it's non–negotiable. He doesn't do anything with the child. Besides, she's a girl and obviously a mother is best qualified to bring her up.

— *I have to stress that you're starting a war. Nothing is easy in a war nor is logical. You have to avoid falling into traps. If he asked to keep the child, let him have her. Don't let on that you want to claim her. If he guesses that is your weak point he will use it to blackmail you. Don't show him your weak points. Turn your heart to stone and prepare yourself for the prospect that he will have your daughter, for a time at least. He is her father after all. You'll see that of his own accord he will send her back to you. Except if he guesses that you are willing to pay the price. Then he'll try to get the most he can out of it. Keep the word 'war' in mind all the time.*

— And lose my daughter?

— *There can be no sentimentality in a war. What's needed is to be methodical.*

— Even concerning my child?

— *Of course. Listen here, to finish with the matter of the child. I have seen from experience that in nearly all divorces the children are in the middle and both sides have a tug–of–war with them, just to hurt the other pay. They will go to any length, although it's not really the children they care about. They just want to win the claim, the war. So if you truly want what's best for her daughter, try not to make her the bone of contention. This is how you should behave: Say "if you want her, keep her. And when you want, perhaps I can have her for a time." Or rather, "it would help if at least at the beginning you have the child." That way you take away the weapon he thinks he has with which to blackmail you. Stay out of the dead end he wants to close you into.*

— So cruelly?

— *You 'ain't seen nothing yet'. The more he realises you're leaving him and especially that you can stand on your own two feet, without him, you must anticipate rabid attacks It's natural that he should want to believe you can't live without him. So he'll try in every way to chuck you down as low as possible. Using every means, dirty as they may be… And I'll tell you something else that happens a lot: in such cases unfortunately the personal environment also plays an important role: his family and friends, even his lawyers. Whomever he tells 'what has happened to him' — because that's how he'll treat it — most of them will give him advice as to how he can hit you and harm you. It seems that's human nature. When watching boxing in the ring they will shout:*

"Hit him with an upper–cut!... get him on the ropes!... knock him out!" It's sad, but people love to see blood. I don't believe that human beings are decent and kind.

I take a deep breath and after a short silence I continued.

–... I believe that when we are born we are like beasts of the jungle: wild animals. Nature has endowed us with aggressiveness and ferocity so as to be able to survive. But a civilised upbringing and education castrates us so that we can live in organised societies, with rules. We are raised to be good workers, to work for the common good – a grandiose task – denying our individuality...

I often employ exaggerated and extreme examples, better to spur on those who seek my advice. I also endeavour to give some philosophical dimension to what I say. I avoid facile preaching or telling them "what to do", of the sort: "you should do this, that or the other", although this is what most people are looking for. They insist, in fact, because it releases them from responsibility for their acts. How many times have I not heard "this is what my mother – or my friends or my psychologist – told me to do."

When I give my views a broader aspect, the patient can, if they agree with them, espouse them too and, through this angle on things, form a personal stance and course of life of their own. It would be a course bearing their own stamp of option, not merely what somebody else indicated. Somebody, who would of course also bear the responsibility for the ultimate choice.

I was trying to put her in the right frame of mind for the fight that goes on in the arena, to prepare her for the war she had started with her husband. I wanted to transmit the message that things would not be easy.

– Even if you sometimes think you are being offered a favourable solution to the divorce procedure, you have always to be suspicious. Don't forget: 'All that glistens is not gold'.

– You make it sound awfully difficult. Are you trying to dissuade me from getting divorced?

– No, of course not, if that is your decision. But I have to prepare you for the worst. I wish such preparation for battle may never be necessary, but remember too the proverb "if you wish for peace, prepare for war", as the ancient Romans said. I don't want you to say after a defeat "I wish I hadn't stated a war." Because, you know, if you are defeated, i.e. if you retreat, afterwards things will be much worse than they are now.

– So what do you suggest I do?

– Be well prepared. That means, to find your husband's weak points before you launch an attack: What his real financial situation is. What he has declared and what he has hidden. Find documentation that could be decisive weaponry for your battle for freedom. An as the ancient Chinese general says in his Art of War: "The enemy must not know your intentions."

– *I never envisaged we would reach this point. But as you say, I was quite right to gather data about his finances and his companies, in which he has not included me anywhere.*

– *So you see, he was getting ready all this time. He made sure you wouldn't have wings to fly away from him.*

Her expression hardened and I saw the decisiveness on her face. A combative frame of mind, as if she was saying "I'll show him!"

I think I had played my role successfully. I had achieved my goal. I felt satisfaction at what I had done. I had transformed a woman from being a victim into a tough fighter with resolve.

I took her to the door. She shook my hand, and I told her I was always there for her. And I left for last the best phrase I use for those who have decided to separate: "It's worthwhile trying to find something else in your life."

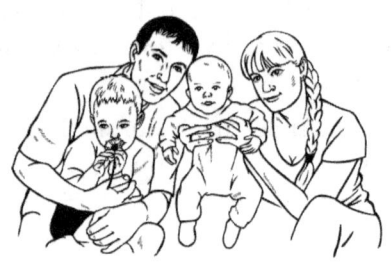

PARENT – CHILD RELATIONSHIPS

I SEE parents in crisis almost every day: Parents who are unsure that they are handling their relationship with their children correctly; Desolate parents, desperately seeking guidelines for the proper method to bring their children up.

There are simple instances, such as traditional families with one or two children, as well as complex situations with children from previous, broken marriages. More or less, in all uncertainties of parents who worry about their behaviour, the guilt predominates in case they are not doing the right thing by their children. Children who may sometimes be over 20 or 30 years old!

The causes are historical here again. Until WWII children were an appendage to a traditional family. The father was the master walking ahead, the wife followed behind, and the children came last. Furthermore, the children followed in a line according to age. Their value in the family framework was according to their rank in the sequence of birth. There was no dispute as to the role each family member played. The parents gave the orders and the children executed them according to the capacity of each.

Whoever felt this framework oppressed them had no choice but to leave. History is full of examples of successful people who left home to try their luck, and distinguished themselves. Most of our national benefactors in Greece quitted their village to chase their dreams in the unknown. Anybody who stayed behind had to obey the strict rules of family and the regional society.

This state of affairs changed after the Second World War. The increase of births of the baby boom, in parallel with the dizzy financial boom suddenly brought children to the tip of the consumerist pyramid. Everything was produced for children; everybody was preoccupied with the children. The Lilliputian consumers became the monarchs of a consumerist society.

At the same time, when the question of nourishment had been solved, Western society turned to psychoanalysis. However, one the main maxims of the theory of psychoanalysis is none else than 'everything is the parents' fault'. In this way parents became the target of all those who promoted themselves in defence of children. Writing, the Press, the radio, television, cinema, everything spoke of the great responsibility of parents toward the vulnerable little beings. Except that the little darlings, if given the opportunity can easily be transformed into little monsters.

This is just what happened. The parents, guilt–ridden by the dominant psychoanalytical theory, are willing, on the one hand, to do everything for their kids, outbidding in the hyper–production of consumer goods and services, while on the other developing an unbounded over–protectionism. Both behaviours, however, proved to be disastrous for both the parents and the children.

Being over–protective not only made for stress and guilt in the parents for fear of giving the children less than they should, it also made for spoiled children. The word 'spoiled' is now in our everyday vocabulary whereas until the mid–twentieth century it hardly existed. Even children born into royal households were brought up in those days extremely strictly. The upbringing of a noble or an aristocrat had nothing to do with what the nouveau–riche of today do for their children. But unfortunately for these parents, this is simply a way of disabling the scions of the financially comfortable bourgeois class.

These children have grown up in circumstances in which they were over–supplied, which is to the detriment of competition. Luxuries are proffered generously and requiring no effort, resulting in the children never learning to fight to acquire them. So, naturally, it is to be expected that when they begin their own life they cannot survive.

It is even more the case in our day, when competition is on a global scale. In agriculture, industry, commerce and services, Internet brings international competition to our door. What consequently will be the fate of a child who grew up over–supplied and over–protected in succeeding to beat one who grew up in penury and for whom the struggle for subsistence is a second skin?

Nowadays in fact, the situation of the spoilt kids of the rich is even more difficult, because even a good education is no longer a prerogative of expensive schools. Education is not for the rich and privileged few alone, since it is accessible on Internet to anyone wanting it, offered for free, without making distinctions.

I often think this when I hear parents confiding their anxieties to me about their children's performance in school:

– *I have got a math tutor for him. And another one for physics and my husband and I do history with him and the other subjects too…*

– *And if you let him manage on his own?*

– *How can you say that, Doctor? What if he had to repeat the grade? He doesn't do his homework on his own…*

– *Oh, do you perhaps also chew his food for him? What do you mean, "he doesn't do his homework on his own"? If he can't do his homework, he ought to stay in the same grade so as better to learn the curriculum. Is it <u>you</u> going to school or he? Isn't it his responsibility to learn what school is trying to teach him so as to be able to function in tomorrow's society? Thank God, you managed to reach this point. You are no longer obliged to get an education.*

– *But Doctor, I'm trying to tell you he doesn't care!*

– *Evidently he thinks his future is assured.*

– *That's easy to say… Nowadays everything can topple over.*

– *Yes, I do know that, but your son doesn't seem to. You have given him a sense of security so it's reasonable that he shouldn't see why he needs to make any effort. That's where you're making a mistake. That's what you should work on: not 'do' his history for him but show him how competitive life is. That's the best thing you can teach him, for him to be motivated to be a good pupil and acquire the equipment necessary for his life.*

– *Yes, I've said just that a thousand times.*

– *And however many times you say it again it will still be no use. Lecturing him is the worst thing you can do for him. Whatever you want to say, to have effect has to be in as indirect manner as possible, for the child not to feel it is being lectured. Children resist to lecturing, especially by their parents. Can't you see that kids have anti–bodies to what parents say? Even before you open your mouth to say something they have already 'protected' their ears from your words.*

– *So how are we supposed to say it?*

– *Talk about it as being about a third person. For instance, how so and so went bankrupt and his children, who grew up in cotton wool now have to find a job. And those poor kids are useless, they don't know how to do anything… If at least they had some sort of diploma, a friend could give them a job in his business. But now what work can he give them to do? Answer the phone, or clean the storeroom? He couldn't do that… And let me tell you, even answering the phone they wouldn't be as good as the very courteous receptionist he has now, nor would they do a better job with the storeroom than the immigrant workers are doing now. As everyone says, now is not a time for acts of charity... They should have been alert... Their parents gave them every opportunity. They went to a good school and the parents helped them in every way as long as they had the financial means to do so. Now it's stormy weather how are they going to survive...?*

— So you too must do your homework...

— No! Wrong! That's the mistake most people make. Let him draw his own conclusions. He's intelligent. Don't rub the conclusion to be made in his face, because then you have achieved nothing. Do as I say... It has to enter his head as an independent piece of information, to make him think, and make a difference to his personal outlook on the world. For it not to be part of his parents' views, which in any case the child doesn't want to listen to.

There are delicate differences in the way we transmit a message, which can completely misrepresent it. What I insist on to all parents is that they have to realise they cannot direct their children. What is easily done is to have them take the opposite direction from the one they wish. Children are vulnerable to every sort of influence except their parents'. They can be influenced by their friends, their teacher, an uncle, a father of a friend, television, any third person but the parent. The parent can influence the child only negatively. That is, to tell it something only to have it do the exact opposite.

If we parents realise this we will comprehend that it needs great mastery to guide a child where we think it ought to go. It requires mastery and strategy. Our moves and our words should not betray our intentions. It is quite a difficult goal for over–protective parents who cannot restrain their anxiety.

— Doctor, he wants to go on a five–day school trip. I can't allow it. The things we hear every year! I don't trust the teachers. What am I going to do if he has an accident?

— Harden your heart. Anyway, pretty soon he'll be going out in the evening and come back in the early hours. He may already be riding a scooter without your knowing. You can't be after him all the time.

— But that's what I want to do.

— If you did and he was aware of it, that's when he would step on it and then... he would surely kill himself.

— That's why I can't help worrying about him all the time.

— You mean, when he starts going out, as is proper, you'll stay awake waiting for him behind the window.

— How can I sleep when my son may be in danger?

— Well, what do you think is achieved by staying awake? All it does is annoy the kid.

Increase the rift between parent and child and may make him come home even later and even more drunk.

– How can you say that? I just want to be close to him all the time, like his guardian angel.

– Yes, but unfortunately you have to realise that despite your good intentions your son sees you not as a guardian angel but rather as... the devil. And your son will see you and want get as far away as possible. And he will be right. His role is to manage to fly alone, with his own wings. Not to stay in the family nest. He must be able to be based on his own powers. Contrary, it would be a problem if he didn't want to leave your side and was comfortable in the nest, fed by the food you provide him with. You too have to realise a parent's role is to show the child how to fly so as later to be able to be admired for flying far and doing great things, on their own.

– And if they can't? We will watch our son breaking his bones and we will stand by and admire?

– Why should he break his bones? Don't you have any confidence in him? You ought, properly, to have taught him to manage, himself. And I'll tell you something else: parents mould a child in the early years of its life. Thereafter they won't change, whatever they do. At any rate they don't change because of the parents' admonishing. Only their experiences change them. So, they have to have as many experiences as possible, positive and negative. It's the only way they will one day be able to stand on their own feet in the difficult world our society lives in. Of course it is expected that children make mistakes, they can't be avoided. It's the mistakes they'll learn from. If at every wrong turn you intervene and straighten the wheel for them they'll never learn to drive by themselves and travel through life.

– And what will the parents do, all alone, once the children have gone?

This came out involuntarily. Perhaps I was expecting just that at the back of my mind. Expecting her to express the anguish most parents have when the children grow up and test their wings. Naturally, I was not going to let this opportunity slip.

– Do you mean to tell me you had your son so that he could look after you in your old age?

– Weeell, not just like that. But won't he be with us? ... Will he throw us out?

– He won't throw you out. He will fly off. You have to stay behind keeping an eye on him. And if he asks for your help, give it to him, if you are able to, of course. Except that's when there'll be a problem with your spouse.

– There will?

– You'll have to learn to live alone, the two of you together. Believe me, it's not easy for a lot of couples.

This is a very common dialogue with parents, and I think it illustrates the dead–end in parent–child relationships in our modern over–protective bourgeois society. A family where the children are the hub around which, besides, most of the aspirations revolve. If Little Georgy is a success, the whole family has triumphed! It is not only the success or failure of the child itself. Because of course the theory of psychoanalysis has convinced everybody that Mummy and Daddy are responsible for Georgy's performance. Not he himself with his brains.

In such cases, my wish for Georgy is that he should rebel and get away as soon as he can. The longer he stays put, the more his wings will be clipped. Furthermore, the worst is that in the end his parents will actually be even more disappointed that their sprout did not manage to fly. So of course, not only will they not stop putting him down, which is what happens when they do not show confidence in him, they will moreover feel remorseful, guilty of having brought up a useless person.

Yet the parent's role is always to teach the child to become self-reliant, or as we say, to paddle his own canoe. This means that the parent ought to create conditions of social competitiveness within the familial greenhouse. Straying behaviour ought to be punished, as it will be in the future, when the child is a member of a cruel society. School too plays a similar role, which is not only to educate but also to teach how to compete.

Let us not forget that behaviour patterns are programmed early in life. Afterwards it is extremely difficult to alter them. If therefore a programme is loaded that says 'never mind if you stole or if you ate the pudding that was for our guests' or '… if you go to school without having done your homework', '… you'll still have your parents' unreserved love and admiration', it is to be expected that such conduct will be repeated later out in the world. Of course, carrying such luggage in their head, they will not be able to understand why society punishes them and marginalises them, since at home they used to be rewarded.

That 'spoiled brat' will therefore have to form new programmes that say that: out in the world different rules apply; that all the old programmes are consequently for home and family consumption alone. But to make new programmes there have to be corresponding social experiences. Certain practices must be condemned so as to be connected to negative sentiments and be scorned. This is however a much harder way to learn than if socially acceptable manners were already learned from the parents and school.

Downgrading: A canker in a relationship

IN A PARENT–CHILD relationship, it happens all the time, the parent is always putting the child down. Rarely does a parent acknowledge the child's worth and, especially, will they show it. From the moment a child is born, a parent will compare it to the next, the sister's, the neighbour's, the teacher's ...the king's little prince. Even worse is when they compare it to the model they had in mind when they had a dream about the family they would have. It must be expected however that no child will ever surpass dreams and myths.

But disdain is the sister of criticism. Wanting our child to be better we keep criticising it and often compare to it to something better:

— *Your little cousin got higher marks than you did…*

So naturally the child answers:

— *Well then adopt her and leave me alone.*

Grown–ups think that criticism will impel a child to do better and sometimes it is true, criticism can become a motivation. But unfortunately most often children will interpret it as disdain, so that instead of trying harder they react in the opposite way than expected.

In fact, if frequently criticised, children feel that there's nothing they can do to please their parents and simply give up trying. They surrender and usually turn to other fields of competition where they think they have a better chance of succeeding. Instead of studying they turn to their gang, scooters, games on Internet or, alas, even to being a 'tough guy', a hooligan, which is the antechamber to narcotics.

A child, and particularly an adolescent, seeks compliments and rewards. These should be given them through the channel of creative activities, else they will be sought in other directions. In simple words, this means parents should reward their children's achievements. Just as they applauded when their child first stood up and took its first steps, they must subsequently show admiration for every effort their child makes:

— *Good for you, Bobby! You know your 2 times table! You'll do it for the 3 times table too. I'm sure you'll do as well further on. Bravo! If you are brave and try hard you can do anything.*

And not:

— *O.k. the 2 times table is easy. It isn't much of a success to know it. Let's see what you do with 3.*

And worst of all:

— *Listen to me, I know it all by heart…*

It may seem like nothing, but it is important. Instead of being coaches, parents behave like opponents. Instead of encouraging, they deprecate. Without being aware of it, as the child grows up they begin to become rivals. Even worse,... but true, to become jealous of it.

What are they jealous of? For one thing: their youth. It is everyone's dream to return to the paradise of youth. Return to the time when responsibilities were light and the struggle was virtual and not the real thing in the social jungle. Return to the days when everything could be excused and nothing was condemned. When punishment was mostly a family affair and not what a faceless society does.

They are even jealous that the child has parents with comprehension, permissiveness and in most instances with more to offer the child than what they themselves had when they were little.

– *We were poor…*

– *Who would have dared to talk back to our parents?*

These comments, so common, conceal a bitterness as well as jealousy. A jealousy that unavoidably later comes out as rivalry; a rivalry that takes the form of strict criticism and downgrading, as well as antagonism that can sometimes not be hidden. I shall never forget how annoyed I was, when I was a young psychiatrist, if my father, also a psychiatrist at the end of his career 'stole' patients from me. This is also why it is extraordinarily difficult for a child to do well in the father's business. The antagonism between the generations cannot be avoided, will come out and poison the relations between parents and children.

The contest of generations

WHO STARTED it, and who was right? I don't think this question makes much sense. Psychoanalysis casts the burden of responsibility on the parents. It demands of the parents to be the most conscientious and therefore the most self–controlled. That, for the parent, means to be the object of their children's expected and normal attacks without reacting.

However, I do not only find this doctrine to be futile, but that it is positively dangerous for the children because, due to this, the children will grow up in a virtual reality. In an environment where there is no rivalry, no clashes nor wars, with the result that they will go out into an unfriendly society unprepared.

The other thing in this dogma I disagree with is that, by the guilty feelings it creates, what it does is to oblige people to hide their intentions. Whilst psychoanalytical theory ostensibly professes the exact opposite, which is to reveal one's innermost intentions, it impels people instead to conceal them better, since those intentions are censured. It adulterates, so to speak, relations among people.

Particularly in the bosom of the family, where guilt feelings circulate, relationships are in the end made more complicated.

And the cherry on the cake of this theoretical approach, made of terms of supposed enlightenment and proclamations on behalf of children's rights, is the absolute condemnation of physical punishment. It would be more hygienic for the relations among the family members if a slap or two were to be administered by the stronger to the weaker, whether between parents and children or among the children. A slap is much preferable to the aggressiveness being transformed into criticism and covert belittling by the one of the other.

We have, sadly, reached the point where what is sought is authenticity. Human relations have lost their immediacy. It is the same with parent–child relations. Anger is cloaked, but so also is love not expressed as it should, in the mistaken fear that it might be misinterpreted. We ought to take a step back in what is wrongly considered the ennoblement of our relationships. We definitely ought to find our genuineness again.

Specifically in regard to parents, I say they need not hide their annoyance when the little one is naughty. Let them yell at the kid, let them mete out some punishment. It doesn't even matter if they hit it, if the former had no effect. It is no crime, nor will it traumatise the child for the rest of its life!

Naturally, I do not mean that excessive and constant violence is justified. In general, the punishment should fit the crime. The principle of equivalence is a basic pillar of justice. Parents should be giving their tots lessons in justice all the time. I say 'the tots' to underline once more that the lessons of essence given by the parents are in the first 3 to 5 years of life. Later than that, the potential for influencing and teaching the young new ways diminishes dramatically. Once the child has formed a personality of its own, it learns almost exclusively from its experiences. As to the parents' teaching, their children become ever less permeable to it, because it should be known that in the process of acquiring an independent identity, children develop anti-bodies to the voice and the admonishments of their parents.

The Rule of Three S

I TELL whoever asks me for a concise formula for bringing up their children about the Rule of the Three S's: Seriousness, Stability and Steadiness.

Seriousness: They must first of all treat their children seriously, as if they were grown-up adults, not like beings who know nothing and have no right to learn the truth about the world. Beings we can fool with fairy tales and lies.

When they discover a lie we have told them, to their eyes the entire structure we have built for them disintegrates in their eyes. Do not forget that the parent's role is to form the child so as to be able to enter society well prepared. There is no point in telling it about mythical situations and inexistent conditions of life. It is besides being dishonest to our children to bring them up in a false world with principles that do not correspond to anything outside the home and the family.

Children have excellent judgment and maturity, far beyond what we can estimate. Remember that in their early years perform enormous progresses. They come into our world knowing nothing and very speedily learn everything. So, it is an error to download false data into their mind's computer. All they will learn is to draw false conclusions. If for instance we teach them that the bad wolf is always punished, in the rest of their life they will expect absolute justice, which is unfortunately something that does not exist.

And something more: whatever we have inculcated at the beginning, in the first years, that also form their scale of values, we must be aware will be difficult to change later. It is the first estimates, the initial evaluations of most of the world's aspects, which constitute the axes upon which children will base themselves for the rest of their life. Thus if for example, just to get their children to eat up they frighten them with 'the bad gypsies who will steal them away' and suchlike imaginary monstrosities, in the future it will be hard for the child to reset this distortion of their convictions about gypsies.

I must have been 6 or 7 when, seeing a splendid car, a Citroen, I told my father how impressed I was. I do not remember whether I said: "Why don't we get one like it?" but what I remember to this day is that he answered – and of course I admired his knowledge of cars – dismissively, "Citroens break down a lot."

Although it was many years ago and I acquired my own knowledge about cars, this comment still influences my preferences. It might have been said flippantly, just to give me an answer rapidly, or to be 'rid' of me at that moment, yet it was printed on my mind for always. Every time it comes up, my father's evaluation is what comes to my mind first and then, in a second stroke, I need to use my logic to cancel it.

This is why I say we have to treat children seriously, as if they were grown–ups.

Stability means we must be stable in what we tell them and what we do to our children. It is not right to forbid something and a little later to permit it. Either because the kid grumbled or cried, or because its friend turned up and we want to seem easy–going and indulgent to a third person, or in the end that we would rather they went off to play and leave us in peace. Such disjointed and uncoordinated behaviour on our part transmits the message to the child that everything is negotiable, that they can reverse our decisions and our rules with diverse strategies.

Successful strategies will be repeated and will become part of the everyday programmes, that is, what we call character, or personality. If for instance they manage to get around us by whining and thus make us change our mind, we should know that in real terms we are encouraging them to complain for the rest of their life. They will try to solve their differences with their future spouse, or boss, or in general whoever they have problems with by grumbling.

It has been proven by experience that children, however small, are terrifyingly strong at getting their own way. They do not give up easily at all. They will cry until they get what they want and are satisfied. From the very first day the baby comes home from the birth clinic it may bawl heartrendingly and for so long that it seems like an age, in order to be fed at the time when it wants. But we must think that in the clinic our baby was being fed at regular hours and that of course none of the nurses in the department for the newborn was in the least touched by the chorus of wails and complaints she was hearing. If we are as consequent in our keeping to feeding times and maintain our steady attitude, then even a baby will manage to adjust its needs to the strictures of its surroundings. If, on the contrary, we rush to give it what it wants every time it cries, the baby will register, inscribed deep in its mind, that it can have what it wants. It suffices to make a lot of noise about it!

Everyone must see that this is the best way to train an anti–social person who in the future will consider the laws of society as being negotiable, as were the family rules at home.

The third rule, that of **Steadiness**, is of course directly related to the foregoing one. If we promise something, either positive or negative, we must be in a position to carry it out. We often say things to children without reckoning on the consequences. We need to be careful about the promises we make to our children, more so even than the promises we make in our professional workplace.

You cannot imagine the depth of a child's disappointment when we have promised we will do something and later do not keep the vow. It is natural that the child should conclude that all the codes and values we have taught it are not consistent in their application and are instead liable to be applied selectively. The entire structure of the child's relations to its environment loses its consistency. Imagine if you were to deposit your monies in a bank because it promised to give you a high rate of interest and, when you went to collect your profit the bank said it could not pay anything! If the cashier said: "That's the way it is… we sometimes promise something we don't really mean. It isn't the end of the world… you're still o.k. ..." I use the words that we adults sometimes use, thinking that we can painlessly extract ourselves from having gone back on our word to the child.

It also often happens that I hear parents threaten their children with the most awful punishments that it is obvious they will never carry out. And I wonder how is it possible that these parents do not see that the only thing they achieve thereby is to lose credibility in their children's eyes? How can a child believe it when in the future they are again threatened with a punishment that the child now knows will never happen? All the parents have done is to make what they say worthless.

This brings us back to Rule One, of being serious. When talking to our children we must treat them as seriously as we would an adult interlocutor, and a stern one at that. Do not airily pronounce things, because that teaches them that everything around is light and easy and that there are no repercussions for what they say or do.

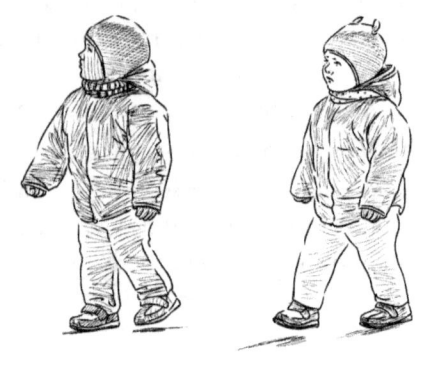

TWO 'LOVING' SIBLINGS

I STILL remember the first time that as psychiatric resident I attended the meeting of the clinical department where I was working. As is usual, the colleague who was responsible for the patient who was admitted to our department for hospitalisation that morning presented the data of his file which he himself had just gathered.

When I heard the patient's family history, I shuddered. Brutal parents who rejected him, hard childhood, traumatic experiences at school and a family stigmatised by the neighbourhood. There followed repeated rejections by the opposite sex and bad professional adjustment. Influenced as I was at the time by the psychoanalytical theories of those days, the first thing that came to my youthful mind was: "With a history like that it was obvious he would fall ill"; "How can anyone survive such psychological stress?"

In the days that followed I heard more case histories until it was my turn to obtain a psychiatric history myself. All the histories contained horrific situations, well out of the ordinary rule that we all know about 'ideal' or 'correct' family relationships. I did not hear of loving, happy parents. Nowhere were there relationships of harmony between parents and children, nor among brothers and sisters. I gradually came to believe that all who came to the psychiatric clinics for help were people from a problematic family background. I found that the other residents had the same conviction, and we shared our qualms.

Until the day came when I imagined myself in my imagination in the patient's place. I wondered what I would tell someone who was taking my family history. What would I say about my parents' relations, their relations with me and my sister as well as mine with my sister? I saw then that there was something wrong with the picture of model family we had been given. I started asking the other residents about their own family history, and we all found, to our amazement, that the world is far from the ideal we thought it was. I anxiously tried to find in my thoughts what family I knew in my milieu that was the ideal: Not one. There is no such thing as the ideal family!

I then realised that all the information we collected from the family history were for the most part superfluous. There is no point in looking in the family closet for its skeletons. Every family has skeletons hidden in the closet, irrespective of the picture it projects. As a matter of fact the guilt we feel for the difference between our family and the ideal one makes us embellish the image of our family. In this way families in our society resemble the saloons of the Far West: they have a fine façade whereas the rest of the building behind is a ruin. From the outside we all see the pristine facades and feel diminished by our own structure, our family and its eccentricities.

As confessors, we psychiatrists have the opportunity to find out was the façade conceals that is all society sees. After so many years practicing my specialisation I am quite convinced that the ideal family we were taught in primary school books is a luminous exception to a rule that in general lines follows the law of the jungle, which is the domination of the strong over the weak. I state my position categorically because I think that in this way I help all those who feel bad because their family does not come under the ideal model considered as the general rule. It is a duty of psychiatry to rid society of distorted convictions that cause more problems than what they try to solve.

I have said all this in introduction to this chapter because the heading 'Two loving siblings' is still contemporary society's greatest taboo. Parents are permitted to quarrel, to be cruel to or neglect their children, but the kids have to be fond of one another. The parents may separate, divorce, form a new family and have more children, but brothers and sisters have no reason not to be loving. They have to love one another and stand up for each other!

There is no greater hoax than this, and the worst of it is that most feelings of guilt are twined into it. Of the siblings themselves, who usually hate and are jealous of their brothers and sisters as well as of the parents who feel at fault for not building loving relationships among their children.

I have heard so many stories about a dying parent's last wish for his children that they should always love one another. There have even been parents who on their deathbed made their children swear their love for their siblings on oath. They feared so much for the destiny of their children's relations to one another after their death that they made them swear, right there in front of them, shortly before their last breath.

This description of scenes so emotionally charged gives an idea of the burden of the sentiments of the taboo of the 'loving siblings', at least on the part of the parents. However, in most cases it is the parents themselves who, consciously or inadvertently undermine the relations among their offspring. The biggest bomb usually lies in the division of the parental property.

I cannot tell you how often I have heard of the breaking up of good or anyway tolerable relations of brothers and sisters after the death of a parent who left some property to his children. And believe me, it is usually not the size of the inheritance that really plays that role. It is simply the real or imagined injustice of the parents that acts as catalyst to the emergence of suppressed feelings of rivalry and consequently the breaking up of the relationship among siblings.

There is one typical instance I remember among many: A woman aged about 50 came to me for help because she was depressed. When I asked her what the cause of her sadness was, she told me her father had died a year ago.

— *How old was your father?*

— 85. *I know, it was time for him to go… and he had had several strokes recently and had been bed-ridden for a year.*

— *However much you loved him, I can't believe that his death is what brought you to this state.*

— *Yes, that's true, it wasn't so much my father's death as how my brothers and sisters and my mother behaved… We have a house in the village, our family home, and my father left it to my little sister.*

— *So what? It was his; he could do what he liked with it. Besides, from what I gather, you don't need an old house in the village. You said your husband is an engineer and has a construction business, and you are a lawyer. You are fortunate that if you wish you can build yourself a country house anywhere you like.*

— *Yes, but I would like my children to be able to go to our village. And moreover my sister doesn't have any children. What will happen to the house? Who will inherit it?*

— *Are you perhaps being a little vindictive?*

— *Oh no, quite the contrary. My sister has formed a camp with my mother and my elder* brother. My other two brothers are on my side and don't speak to Mother and the other two.

— Just a minute. From what I understand you are five brothers and sisters. Three boys and two girls.

— That's right. My brothers got their share from my father, for their businesses. He had given them land and money when they needed it. So now they had no rights to a share of the house and the field which was all that was left. But the eldest brother persuaded our mother to give me the field and the house to my sister. Why?

— Is your younger sister perhaps be more in need than you?

— It isn't my fault if that's what she made of her life. But she was always in cahoots with our older brother. And she was always Mother's favourite. It was Mother who spoiled her chances, being over protective, and my sister never married. Nobody was good enough for her. Our mother made a snob of her and there you are, that's the result. She is alone... Now she can jolly well take care of Mother in her old age.

— So you see: crime and punishment. What do you care, though? Let them stew in their own juice. The best punishment is to be magnanimous.

— That's what my husband says too. But I can't see it that way. I'm infuriated. I had been rid of my sister and her manipulations of my mother. Now my father's will, has brought it all back up to the surface.

— Who was your father's favourite child?

— Me, of course. That's why I was so hurt. They found him, my mother specially, when he was weakened and they made him draw up that unfair will...

Alliances are formed in every family. Most common are father and daughter on the one side and mother and son on the other. But let us not forget that when we speak of alliances, it is war we're speaking of. We mustn't ignore the fact that in every family there are rivalries. As a rule, the parents' rivalry is transferred to the children, generally in the form of alliances. How often have I not heard the words: *"My husband (or my wife) turned the children against me"*!

It is standard for children to utilise the contention between parents and therefore to be expected that fronts will be put up among the young. Between those children who have one parent as a model, and the others, who admire, and perhaps imitate, the other: The boys against the girls or the younger against the elder. And of course, any other combination is also possible.

A further factor that frequently plays a big role in intra–family relations is the one of strength. A parent often favours the one they consider to be the weakest. However, strength and forces are not always real. Many children, so as to get their parents' cherishing 'play' the weak one. They do not really lack strength but they have learned early in life that when they fall and hurt themselves, the mother or the father stopped playing with another child and rushed to see to the one who was hurt. Very reasonable, you will say. But quite a lot of children found this was the 'button' that triggered the attention of a parent.

We have to thing generally, of the ways in which each child tries to capture the interest of the people around it. If one child was well–behaved, the other can be expected to be naughty. If one child runs off to the left and the parent chases after it, the other will go to the right to grab the attention of the parent. If in fact it doesn't see any reaction from the parent, it will start screaming or grizzling or will fall down and hurt itself!

I tell all the parents I see that their children are tougher than they think, and they are also a kind of 'perverse'. They have no compunction to do things that adults find incomprehensible. They can easily sob with such passion and intensity, so heart–rendingly, that they sound as though they are being slaughtered. They can vomit their favourite food or not play with their favourite toy so as to alarm their mother, who will be afraid that 'something has happened to the child'. Kids will often pretend to be afraid of the dark so as to go crying to their parents' bed and not allow their new–born sibling to monopolise the parents' bedroom.

They may start wetting themselves, like the baby, to show they have the same needs as the baby. However familiar this symptom may sound, it does require complete suspension of inhibitions as well as 'perversity' of mind to be achieved. Think how hard it is for an adult to wet their bed on purpose. Children however are not put off by such details. How decisive they are in capturing the interest of parents is truly limitless.

It is worth thinking about what a shock it is to a child when a baby sibling is born. It suddenly realises that someone else has entered his space and gains a portion of what is most valuable: the love and attention of the most important persons in the world. Whereas until just recently it was the epicentre of its whole world, now it sees that all eyes are on the new arrival.

It is consequently understandable and reasonable that the child should do anything in its power to regain what was lost. It is also to be expected that it would wish the intruder out of the way. I say that too straight out, because many siblings have guilt feelings about having such sentiments. They are not few who confessed, fearfully, that there have been moments in their life when they realised they wished the little sibling would die.

Some parents too have confided to me, horrified, that for instance they heard one child asking Santa Claus to take the other child away with him! Such wishes as well as such acts are not rare. The great Italian film director Fellini has an illustrative scene in his autobiographical film Amarcord: a little boy tries to crush his baby sibling, oblivious in its cradle, with a huge rock that he can barely lift!

So, there is no reason to feel guilt for similar thoughts, of one's own, or of our children. They are absolutely normal and expected. It is an obligation for psychiatrists to relieve these people from their unreasonable guilt feelings. We must never forget that the relationship among siblings is always one of rivalry. It is as though there were two or more shops with the same wares in one quarter, addressing the same clientele. Siblings will compete to capture that clientele, in the same way as those shops are, as they try to have their parents' exclusive love and care.

We have to admit that in our modern post–Freudian society, a society of equality and condemnation of repressed emotions, family situations are more complicated. We have dissolved the conventional framework of familial values and traditions because it was 'unjust' and led to inequalities. We gave the two sexes equal status and have in fact recently tried to completely eradicate the differences between them in the game of human relations. That is why it is not strange the see a dramatic increase in homosexuality in our societies.

Therefore, bearing this 'politically correct' model in mind, we try to keep an equal distance from our children. We are not permitted to have a favourite. It is also prohibited for the child to answer the question often posed: "Whom do you prefer, your father or your mother?" The same goes for the parent, who must remain unbiased.

It is here however that the devil lurks. In those objective equal distances, that can never be so. For it is unnatural. Nothing in nature has absolute equality. As long as there are the tiniest differences there will be protests. From the chocolates that have to be divided into equal portions up to the parental property. This is of course irrespective of gender, age and character. It means that a parent, according to the rules of our society, has to keep an equal distance from the good and well–behaved child as from the 'difficult' and naughty one.

According to the social precepts of equality a parent cannot favour the child who indulges them, the one who is no trouble, who does its homework. They are also not allowed to punish the disobedient one. In fact, this attitude of society provides the unruly child with justification for its behaviour, precisely because it is 'unfairly treated'! For parents can of course not act like machines. It is unavoidable that it should escape them from time, to time to show one child some displeasure and some favour to another.

In pre–Freudian days intra–familial relations were simpler. There was punishment, and the naughty one knew very well what it was being punished for. Also, because there were no social inhibitions, punishment was administered with immediacy and was actually very effective. Punishment was moreover of greater pedagogic value, because everybody else knew that if they did something like it they would be punished. Parents were not 'under obligation' to restrain their irritation, nor to be equidistant from their offspring. Rules were simple and directly applicable.

But, 'equal distance' and 'equality' strangled the authenticity and the immediacy of relations within the family. Now, before expressing what they feel, before showing disappointment or admiration, they have to measure whether the first may bother the one addressed, as much as the other the remaining children. We have reached a point where it is a problem to reward one child in case it is misconstrued by or 'upsetting' for the other!

It must also not be forgotten, that in the days of 'inequality' of relations there were clear rules regulating intra–familial relations. Rules nobody could dispute, because they were the laws of custom and respected by all. There were the well-known rights of primogeniture. The first–born had a special position, as did boys who had one place and girls another. Their roles were absolutely distinct and society permitted no margin for contestation.

From a purely psychiatric angle, those socially defined relations were greatly less mentally wearying, than those of modern times that need constant alertness and constant negotiation. In the example I mentioned of the daughter who became depressed after her father's death, because she felt she had been wronged by her mother and younger sister in the matter of inheritance for instance, the law of custom gave clear solutions. Primogeniture in fact, which accompanied humanity for generations, passed paternal property to the first–born so as not to split the property. There was then no question of siblings quarrelling over 'half a field'.

Doubtless, the law of custom may appear unacceptable in the society of our day, but the freedom that has been granted us ought also to bear human frailties and human particularities in mind. The quest for complete equality leads to suppression of emotions as well as to a 'haircut' of the peculiarities of each separate human entity.

I think it indispensable, to enrich the game of our relationships with all those diverse elements of liking and disliking each of us harbours about others: Without concealing them or suffocating them. A girl gives other joys and is otherwise sweet than a boy. A baby has different needs and gives other pleasures than the teenager. It is not bad for anybody to express the corresponding feelings, as long as they are genuine. Let us not put the brakes on them. Let us acknowledge each person's particular needs, but let us also be prepared to be aware of the rivalry inevitable between people. It is impossible to erase this competition and also, not to respond to it.

It is inhuman to demand rivals to love one another. It is like asking them to put aside their feelings and be transformed into machines that compete. Only robots do not hate their fellow robots in a competition. We humans, fortunately, develop feelings regarding our competitors. It is thus human nature that makes siblings not 'loving'. If therefore we require it of them, it is like asking them to renounce their nature and suppress their emotions. It is in essence one more castration by parents of their children. And it is required of parents, who in turn, were emotionally castrated by their parents.

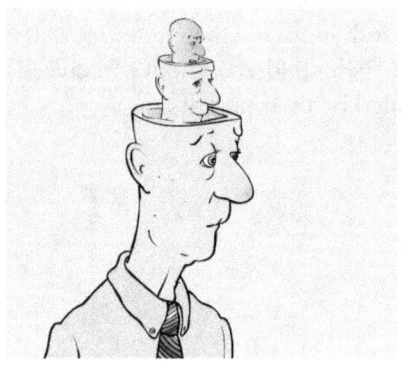

PEOPLE'S PERSONALITY

WHAT MAKES people different is not their appearance but mainly their character, what in psychiatry we call personality. It is the manner in which they respond to the diverse stimuli they receive. Whilst each person's appearance is unique, personalities are in common for huge numbers of people. Someone may be white or black or yellow, tall, short, fat or thin, blue–eyed, auburn, blond, dark, hairy, hairless or bald, squint–eyed, with a crooked nose or flap–eared, but their personality is between two poles: between hysteric and obsessive – compulsive!

I had the good fortune to have as a teacher at the beginning of my training in Psychiatry, one colleague who gave particular weight to the personalities of patients. Besides psycho–pathology, this excellent psychiatrist was also interested in personality, upon which the illness 'sat'. He showed us persistently, how personality colours the manifestation and the symptoms of mental illness.

In fact he encouraged us to study the diverse types of personalities because, he said, such knowledge would arm us with powerful equipment for our everyday relationships. It is true that if you can understand the type of personality of the person opposite you, it is much easier to handle them and direct them where you wish. Since you can foresee their reactions, you know ahead of time what you must say and what to expect from them.

Defining another's type of personality, gives a strong advantage since you are not fooled by the tricks the other has learned to utilise so as to conceal his intentions. Also, knowing their personality you know their mental and emotional needs. You know how you can get close to the person and overcome the defences that they usually employ. You can also estimate what they want from you and how your answer will be taken. In a word, delving into the wonderful world of personality types is an excellent way to be equipped in competitive everyday life.

After this introduction you may think a chapter on the types of personality is very difficult for you to understand, because they are not many who are knowledgeable about it. But the mistake most people make is not to give any importance to the personality of the persons they are in touch with. In this way they are misled by the surface picture and neglect the essence. In the daily struggle most people have learned to give importance to the weapons and armour of the fighter they have opposite them and not to their mind. But, it is the mind that will give the command for the direction and the use of the weapons. We should therefore concentrate on our opponent's mind. How it will function depends above all on their personality.

People's personality, however, does not at all have the uniqueness you might expect. The number of scenarios is extremely small and moves between two poles. At the one end is what we in psychiatry call a hysterical personality; and at the other what we call obsessive –compulsive. Be careful though, the use of such terms in this context is different from what most of the people think and does of course not suggest the existence of any mental disturbance. It is perfectly healthy to have either a hysterical or an obsessive–compulsive personality, to be one or the other. We all of us besides, have some elements of these two extremes. We are all somewhere between the two.

Hysterical personality

I HAD a friend, named Amalia. She is a successful notary, married, with two grown children. At whatever event she sees me she greets me from afar and comes over to give me a big hug. She kisses me on both cheeks, careful not to mess her makeup, of which there is always quite a lot. She speaks loudly, using exaggerated adjectives and superlatives wherever she can:

– Yesterday we went to an extraordinary place. You've never seen such beautiful surroundings and... let me tell you, 'la tout Athènes' was there!

She will use foreign expressions wherever possible, never mind if not always correctly. What matters for Amalia is the pronunciation. I have to say it is faultless in all languages. She can, you see, imitate absolutely convincingly. She is an actress and thinks she is on a stage all the time.

– ... *Only you were missing. Next time I go, we'll make arrangements to go together. With your wife of course! Where is the sweet thing? I don't see her...*

She is constantly looking around, seeking out new 'prey', as I put it. She examines who is nearby and whether they are noticing her. I am sure that even if she is kissing her companion on the mouth she does not look at him. Her eyes and her concern are always turned onto the onlookers. It is as if she depended on their applause.

– *And you, you are looking great today.*

– *Why, don't I usually?*

I love to tease her. She is quick–witted and gives as good as she takes in a way of her own, never nasty. She is intelligent and is aware of her 'problem'. She knows she cannot control this entire theatrical element which is how she behaves. She enjoys it and is also pleased when I stress it with my teasing.

– *Of course you do, but today you are glowing. As if you've been having Botox.*

– *My plastic surgeon is more generous. He gives me another ten years before starting a treatment.*

– *You don't say! Everyone starts at 30 nowadays. My dear, all the women here tonight have injections every six months. We two are the only exceptions!*

She laughed loudly and looked around to see if she had been noticed. She always exaggerates, even when it is a serious matter. I have sometimes had to correct her as when for instance introducing me to eminent persons she gave me scientific qualifications and family titles I do not possess.

– *This is how we hysterics are, always a little over the top.*

– *I understand that, but some things can't be inflated. They can't be stretched, however much you would like to.*

– *My love, that's how it is. I live in exaggeration. It's not only that I see everything intensified, my brain too multiplies it all.*

Amalia and I have common friends and I have spoken to them about her. Most of them cannot realise that exaggeration is a characteristic of her personality and therefore they even think of her as a liar. As far as they are concerned anything she tells them is totally unbelievable: "You have to discount whatever Amalia says by half", is what they maintain. Some in fact doubt her systematically, so that they are no longer friends. It is a shame, because she is not a bad person, nor are the fibs told with any particular objective or does she expect any profit from them. It is simply her character and whatever is said to her will not change her. The only thing achieved is that she will dislike them. I, on the contrary, try as much as possible not to correct her and that is why she is so fond of me. I do not flatter her, quite the opposite, we two have had sincere and serious talks about her 'problem'.

Amalia's father was an honest and good accountant. He worked in a major company all his life but, because he was overly honest, never managed to get to top management. So not only did he not make money when he had the opportunity, such as during the war and the German occupation, but in the end the people who managed the company he worked for sacked him because he refused to cover their illicit practices.

So when Amalia was a little girl she experienced the trauma of her family's financial ruin. Child as she was, she despised her father and took charge of her own life. She went 'on stage' and played a role that of course she knew then to be completely false. Already in Primary School, she wrote very imaginative essays. She tried, by the way she dressed or moved or spoke, adding an accent of exaggeration, to show she was something superior to what she really was. Evidently, this succeeded in the circle of her schoolmates and teachers. She lived in an unreal world. But playing the role all the time, she ended by believing it. She became what in the language of the theatre is known as a character actress.

Nevertheless, she is always haunted by the knowledge that it is all a sham. Now she does not have much opportunity to think about it, obviously she avoids doing so, but we have talked about it together quite often. She is aware that all this display is false and that besides it is not her real self. Deep down, Amalia is actually a rather shy and extremely insecure little girl. She has however made a religion of her need to survive and have the affirmation of others. She lives to be applauded. She is why she does everything to be applauded and admired by others. She flatters people she is essentially indifferent to.

She is indifferent to all of them! Yes indeed. Amalia is interested only in herself. She acts a part for the applause. She does not have an emotional relationship with anybody. Not on stage, nor in the stalls. Even her children are an adjunct to her image. That's how she views them. She wants them beautifully dressed, doing well in school and to hear nothing but praise for them. Her children are for her something, like her earrings.

However, from a teenager her daughter threw out the expensive clothes her mother bought her and now dresses only in rags. Her hair is always a mess and she keeps company only with various marginal types. Initially, Amalia told whoever asked her about her daughter that she was having her rebellion. Later on, she decided she could no longer stand it and now does not speak about her daughter at all. As if she did not exist.

Fortunately she has a son who justifies her. He does everything his mother tells him to do to the letter and has become an element of 'good society': Excellent studies, expensive clothes and car, going out with girls with well-known names. He is fulfilling his mama's dream.

And Amalia's husband? As any psychiatrist could foresee, he resembles her father: Colourless, timid, absent from the stage. Amalia is on it alone. She uses him too as a prop. She brings him out when she thinks it serves the purpose of the 'performance'. His personality, it would, is the exact opposite of Amalia's.

To some who stand at a distance, Amalia seems a monster, false, and perhaps finally wicked. I however can assure you that Amalia has given me more than what I have offered her, and with all her heart, simply because I do not react in the same way as most people around her.

I do not focus on the false picture she projects but see deeper, to the need she has to project it. I can safely say I like her, knowing what she hides under all the gestures she makes. Not that I pity her. You should know that hysterical people are very good at communicating sentiments. Emotionally, they communicate more and are consequently good at reading feelings. That way they instantly detect feelings of rejection that often, despite their valiant efforts, appear in others. Amalia could therefore immediately trace the slightest sign of pity in my expression, so I am particularly careful. In my inner self I have besides evaluated that in her way, with this personality, Amalia has succeeded in whatever she has achieved. She is in consequence not to be pitied.

On, the other hand, I can perfectly well defend myself from Amalia's fiery persona. I am not taken in by her intense emotions because I know very well that however positive they might be at one moment they can become just as negative the next, by a mere change of current. Just because something passed through her mind that can better serve her purpose. That is why with Amalia one has at all times to be on one's guard. On the other hand not be disparaging, as are some of those who know her, who of course are also right. One must not be critical, because Amalia senses it straight away which, let us not forget, is particularly painful for such a person.

It is more or less in this way that hysterical people make friends who however alas later become 'enemies'. Or rather, initially people are impressed and want to approach. They are caught by the bait. They are attracted by the constant emotional attacks hysterical persons make all the time. But then many are not able, or not willing, to appreciate them as a whole and, disappointed, they keep their distance. When this takes place often however things get sour, and some friends become enemies. Because, you see, hysterical people cannot in the least tolerate rejection.

When friends and enemies are weighed, in the balance I think the hysterical are the losers. Although they are incredibly able to make friends, they lose most of them. Because, the more enthusiastic the friends are the more they are disappointed and from the friends' camp go over to the enemy. For the hysterical project their emotions but do not really have sentiments. Sentiments are their 'bait' but they cannot really give emotional contact, because 'the Emperor isn't wearing anything at all!'

They are incapable of loving anyone but themselves: Egotists? Maybe. But they do not keep sentiment for themselves. They simply do not have any. Despite their flaming exterior emotional surface, at the core they are, sadly, frozen. The more they are aware of their frozen core, the more they try to project a burning surface, so as to conceal the essence of their existence.

A further tiny characteristic I have observed in many hysterical persons is that they close their eyes when they are speaking. They either lower their lids or turn the irises up so that only the white of the eye is visible. I mention it here because at that moment I feel as though those people are trying to hide their expression. To hide what they feel.

Well, I am very fond of my friend Amalia. I try to assure her of my liking, while at the same time that I do not need her demonstration of affection or sentiments in general on her part. This stance gives her security and with me she opens up, becomes more human. It may be to me alone that she has confided the terror she feels when she realises how cold she is basically.

Hysterical persons are cold in every sector. Sexually, too. They can of course pretend, to perfection, but cannot hide it from their self. That is their tragedy, particularly when their pretence fools the others. Then they are even more scared. They think: "Just imagine if I couldn't put on an act! Everybody would have rejected me and abandoned me." That is why they play their role without respite, while knowing very well that it is not their true self.

The needs for reassurance are great and constant. Because I know this, whenever I can I try to give her something. Whether a glass of water or a glass of wine at a reception, or a flower or gift of a trifle. I know that whatever I offer will be accepted with immense gratitude. And it is certain it will be reciprocated to a multiple degree.

Also, Amalia needs someone to accept her necessities and the rules followed by her mind. She is tired of all those, who with the best intentions, try to put her right. She is tired, for example, of those who comment on her lateness for appointments. She knows they are right, since she is never on time, but this 'habit' is something she herself cannot handle. She has told me that when she is in front of the mirror trying on clothes she feels she is acting, and loses the sense of time. It must be said on the other hand that she is always beautifully dressed. Amalia is never seen badly dressed. Everything about her appearance is cared for to the last detail.

When her husband complains to me, I say:

– I can see you're proud of the way your wife looks, it should be obvious it also has a cost. Instead of pressing her to hurry up because you'll be late for an appointment, relax and think that where you're going everyone will envy you.

– But I can't always be in a rush so as not to be late for something.

– Right, but by pressing her all you do is irritate her and she will take even longer. And then you leave home quarrelling despite going out to have fun.

– Oh, but I haven't told you the worst part. Wherever we arrive late… she always makes sure to say it was my fault.

– That's the cost of accompanying a diva.

But this is the way it is with all people. On the one hand they want to conquer the princess but as soon as they have, they make her clean the grate, like Cinderella. What attracted them, the appearance, the intelligence, the personality… eventually annoys them. To be fair, it is the same for women. They are charmed by the charmer but they then want him to renounce his charm. And of course if he does make the mistake and renounce it, which is to say, to adapt to their framework, then, how strange, he bores them because now, naturally, he is no longer charming.

It is the permanent tragedy of human relations. We are attracted and charmed by what we do not have. Whatever seems exotic to us, the opposite of our own character, far from our usual habits, our own everyday. But it is to be expected, that something like that should delight us at the start and later on is tiresome. We seek to return to our habits, which ensure a smoother and less 'costly' way of life.

This is the point on which most couples clash. Hysterical people charm us but, it is very difficult to put up with them for long. Those who bound themselves to them have a reaction. Those who married one, had children, made a family or even set up business together. Then most of them cannot bear the tendency of hystericals to be always on front stage. And so it is natural they should try to switch roles.

What is contradictory, as well as tragic at the same time is that if after a lot of pressure and struggles the hysterical person gives up their typical manifestations, they automatically lose their charm and the interest they succeeded. And so, the companions and colleagues of hysterical people are disappointed in them and look for fresh emotions, eventually from other hystericals!

If the preconditions and the objective potential exist such a vicious circle may be repeated. Until somebody realises the paradox of human relations: a person looks for something that does not suit them. They are enchanted by what is different from them and their character. But it is not a being that can be lived with. They are people with whom cohabitation is a constant struggle for domination.

I have often been puzzled by this paradox. What I think is that this trend of human beings to seek out what is different is inherited from their animal ancestry. I think, that is, that in animals, evolution engraved in their mind the tendency to seek out something different from them. Nature in this way blends diverse genes, makes new DNA cocktails. Evolution hopes in this way to create new species that might lead to improved editions of living beings.

The calm monkey is attracted by the nervy one, and vice versa. So they copulate, exchange DNA, and other pass the same way. In animals there is not usually any cohabitation of parents. Whenever it is indispensable it will last for a few months at most until the offspring can be independent. No long–lasting cohabitation is required as in the patriarchal human society.

Even in the primitive matriarchal society the men fertilized the women who had selected them, without there being a close relation of living together. All the men were hunters and hunted together, while the women stayed at home and cared for the children, also together. It can be seen that in such a society difference was sought and gave advantages to some in the quest for a sexual partner.

It must be a remnant of this search for the different that makes dark–haired men attractive to blonde women and, contrarily, blond men to dark–haired women. Nature seeks the crossing of different genetic materials. Let us however not forget, that in the example of the blonds and pale–skinned fair–haired they do not do well in places with very strong sun. So although they are desired by the dark–haired, they cannot live with them for very long under the sun!

Compulsive personality

AMALIA'S HUSBAND george, who as has been said, resembled her father, has exactly the opposite type of personality from his wife. He is a civil engineer. When Amalia met him he was still at university. He was in his last year of civil engineering studies and Amalia, who was always ambitious, had plans for a future collaboration. John would build houses and Amalia, who would become a notary, would draw up the contracts.

Although Amalia did become a notary, George, who had done well in his studies, when he graduated however realised he was not made for entrepreneurship in construction. He was incapable of taking a risk. Despite Amalia's urging – who had married him in the meanwhile – he knew it was beyond his powers to negotiate with the land owners and get a loan from a bank. In the first and only attempt he made, he was incapable of bargaining over the exchange partnership. Then when he was told the terms of the loan he could not sleep for two nights. He fidgeted all night, worrying whether he would be able to repay it.

In his mind he imagined all the negative scenarios, even the most improbable: "Supposing I don't sell any flats? If the people I sell to turn out to be unreliable and do not pay me?" The scenarios became even more unlikely as the night went on. "What if I commit some offence of city planning regulations and get caught? And if the owner of the land or some buyer presses me to commit some such offence?" In the morning, as you can imagine, he was a wreck and he announced to Amalia that he was not cut out for such work.

So he preferred to do construction static calculations for buildings. He started an office and did structural calculations for major projects. He was very good at his work and conscientious, and the business was doing exceptionally well. George was in his element. In his work everything was pre–planned, within rules and frameworks. Nothing was left to chance. He did not need any imagination. He could never have worked at something that was based on imagination and initiative. It was enough for him that one plus one should make two. He could not bear imprecision. Already from high school, whilst Math and Algebra were his favourite subjects, he had never liked either fantastic numbers (for him, 'numbers' are great songs), nor the theory of chaos.

Literary writing was always his weak point. He could not let his imagination roam and take him to fictional situations. He is a pragmatist in the extreme. He is very good at descriptions and can elaborate details. But he cannot inject any sentiment, even in his descriptions. It seems that sentiment is an unknown notion for George. He never expresses any sort of emotion. He tries to analyse everything by the process of logic. Even when he speaks he sounds monotonous. His voice is toneless. I have never heard George tell a joke or a story. Once or twice when he tried to tell a story or about some incident from his life, Amalia interrupted him and continued for him. True, the way George tells something is boring to say the least, whereas on the contrary when Amalia talks about something, however trivial, she knows how to do it in such a way that everyone hangs on her lips.

Hysterical persons become the centre of a group while the compulsive are usually in the background. They dare not crack a joke, or if they do they ruin it. The hysterical on the other hand act the parts required by the story–telling. They are in the skin of the characters of the story they are telling. They have a lively way of speaking. Hysterical people steal the show with only a few words, while the compulsive are still thinking about it and trying to evaluate the pros and cons of their participation in the performance.

It is a fact that George finds it very difficult to make any decision. He is the exact opposite of his wife, whose decisiveness is almost impulsive. The result is that they do whatever Amalia wants, simply because George has not had time to decide. While George is still investigating the proposals of friends regarding their summer holiday, Amalia has already booked the tickets.

Chatting with George one day, I mentioned an example I give my students. When I was seventeen I was very anxious and worried about which path I should follow. Should I try to enrol in medical school and become a doctor like my father, or become a car mechanic, an idea that attracted me at the time? It was because I spent a lot of time in a car repair shop where my father used to take our car. I was impressed by their machines and their tuning, which I had begun to learn. At the time, to make a choice of career was a tall order!

Well, now after so many years, I think that on whatever road I had chosen, I would have had more or less the same success. Success and satisfaction do not depend on one option but on each person's resolve to chase after it and fight for it. It was my way of showing George that he need not waste time and his brain's grey matter in making a choice of a decision but in making it materialise.

I knew, of course, that it is difficult for a person to change. A being's personality is like the computer's keyboard. The keys are arranged according to their frequency of use. Those used most often are accessibly in the centre and those least often are in the corners.

As has been said, the brain has flexibility and is capable of altering its connections. At the beginning of life each brain arranges its own keyboard according to the uses made of it. This is the original disposition which is then followed for the rest of life. That is, each person has an accessible repertoire of reactions to specific stimulations. A powerful motive is required and a great effort has to be made in order to change our manner of reacting. It is feasible of course, for the brain remains flexible, but we should be aware that any change becomes more difficult to make as we grow older.

I therefore did not expect George to change, for he did not besides have a strong motive. For one thing, in himself he believes he is always right and that Amalia is simply superficial. I cannot entirely disagree with this. Furthermore, George, a consistent compulsive is particularly inflexible. He does not easily change his ideas and his views on anything. Once something is fixed in his mind it is impossible to persuade him otherwise. If he likes somebody he will continue to do so, whereas if he takes a dislike to someone from the start, it is extremely difficult for him to change his opinion.

This inflexibility of sentiments of the compulsive person is the result of the enormous insecurity they have in dealing with their sentiments. Whilst hysterical are masters in management of sentiment, compulsives get a zero in that chapter. It is exceptionally difficult for compulsives to acquire emotional contact, as it is for them to express their emotion. This is besides why they give the impression of lacking any sentiments.

Just as for hysterical persons however, in the compulsive the surface is misleading. As has been said, because the hysterical know they have a frozen core, they present an outer aspect full of intense, fluctuating emotion, trying to camouflage the problem they feel they have. On the contrary, in the same way compulsive people are really trying to conceal their intense emotions under a stony surface.

That there is so much emotion in the inner core of their existence frightens those with compulsive personalities. They feel vulnerable and try to protect themselves. They freeze their emotional expressions and reactions to such an extent, that they give the impression they have none. But, these tactics finally make them lose the capacity of exploring the sentiments of others. As they grow older, compulsives thus lose any possibility of emotional contact and verbal give and take. The language of sentiment gradually becomes a dead language for them, unknown and useless. In fact, to escape from the difficulties they think an emotional communication has, they concentrate with everything they have on the language of logic.

This is why at school George preferred mathematical calculations to declaring sentiments in an essay. Amalia once showed me copybooks from George's primary school with his essays. On nearly all the teacher had written, in red, "too dry!" In maths however it was always "well done!"

Little did he know then that ten years later he would dare to transgress by approaching the emotional steam–roller that was Amalia! It was inevitable that from the moment George permitted it and became Amalia's target, the outcome was predetermined. Compulsives are charmed by the facility with which hysterical people manipulate sentiment. This is also why they are always shielded of a cold emotional surface: Because they are afraid of being hurt emotionally. It seems though, that at some point Amalia managed to make him feel safe and to loosen his protective measures. She therefore invaded his vulnerable emotional core with her flaming surface and made him her slave forever. He ran after her, and is still doing it, as much in love with her as ever, and much as he may grumble about her 'lateness' and her 'superficialities' he is still attracted to her.

However unsuited they may be, it may be said they have harmony. The one complements the other. When I say harmony, I do not mean in their looks, because goodness knows, as stylish as Amalia is, so colourless is George. Hysterical beings dress vividly, imaginatively, whilst compulsives are conservative, and if they find a style that does not expose them nor betrays them, they stick to it and stay that way always. I say betrays them because basically they are charmed by those who are able to transgress. It is just that compulsives are so insecure that they cancel any flight of their imagination.

All human beings dispose of a personality between Amalia's and George's personalities. On the path, that is, that unites a hysterical personality with the compulsive. In fact most of us have elements from both extremes in our personality. We consist of a mosaic of hysterical and compulsive elements which as a whole result in our being more hysterical or more compulsive types.

If someone investigates the tendency of the sum of our elements, more will be found of the one or the other personality that might not be evident. They will in this way be able to anticipate our reactions and consequently also guide us in the direction they desire. It is therefore worthwhile to explore the personalities of those we are interested in. We will on the one hand find the 'buttons' so as to handle them better and on the other also better be able to manage our relationship with them.

Finally, an interesting observation is that the characteristics of personality can be decisive in our choice of career. For example, a compulsive personality will not succeed in commerce where everything is fluid and negotiable. Their need for stability and clear signals based on objective and measurable values would better suit them to a career in science. In contrast the hysterical personality who easily expresses their emotions and can negotiate anything with outstanding success, would do well in business.

Therefore, one's personality can be crucial in the choice of career, either as a 'merchant' or as a 'scientist'. For example, a merchant would be comfortable in the notion that an ounce of gold can be bought or sold at whatever negotiated price without it being considered a scam, but for the scientist, the exact weight of the gold in relation to the price is crucial.

With this double logic there are people who are either 'scientists' or 'merchants'. In other words, some people move within clearly defined boundaries, while others believe that everything can be negotiated according to their wishes. This is the essential difference—the polarization—that motivates all our personalities.

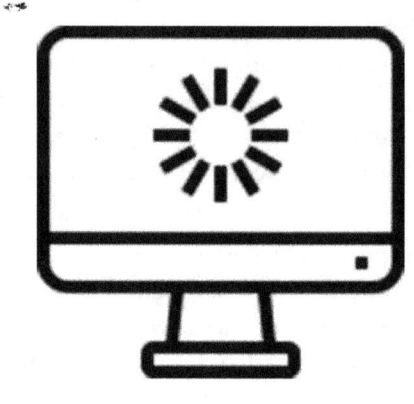

THE DELAY IN PSYCHIATRY

THE GREAT breakthrough in Medicine began at the end of the nineteenth and the first half of the twentieth centuries, with discoveries about anatomy, the relationship between diseases and bodily trauma, and the new knowledge that bacteria and viruses were responsible for a great range of ailments and syndromes. All this made it possible for doctors, who were always looking for the causes of disease, to treat them with scientific accuracy.

Within a few decades, Medicine was able to control most of the spectrum of known conditions with the aid of antibiotics and vaccines. With these basic tools at their disposal, doctors after WWII were able to escape their association with shamans, wizards, and charlatans, and become instead, scientific technocrats whose word could now be trusted almost without question.

Instead of leeches and enemas, there were prescription medicines whose effectiveness had been proven within stringent scientific guidelines. As for the many ailments where a means of addressing their causes had yet to be found, the symptoms could now be dealt with by excising the damaged tissue, even from a distance, under strictly hygienic conditions so as to limit damage to the surrounding tissue.

In the twentieth century we are right to claim a true medical revolution. Medical discoveries used in the economically developed world have extended the average life expectancy to the point where man can arrogantly flirt with the notion of living for more than a hundred years. It is true that in the twenty-first century we have become extremely demanding of medicine. We expect immediate and painless relief of all symptoms, and refuse to excuse the 'failure' of the doctor in providing for our often-excessive requests. It is now difficult for us to accept infirmity or death, and we no longer consider the latter a certainty, but rather a medical error.

However, despite this explosion of medical knowledge, Psychiatry has lagged behind. Of all the known psychiatric conditions, dissection of the brain has revealed lesions only in syphilis, specifically from the later stages, known as Neurosyphilis, when the syphilis bacteria attack the brain. Historians claim that a large proportion—as much as 30%—of inmates in mental facilities in the early twentieth century, suffered from this condition. Symptoms included delusions of grandeur, with sufferers claiming to be kings, nobles, or generals. These were the people who provided society's archetype for the definition of the word 'crazy'.

However, Medicine could find no specific brain damage to explain schizophrenia or the entire spectrum of mental disorders. No autopsy on the brains of dead patients yielded a single abnormality, anatomical anomaly, germ or virus, to explain the symptoms.

Freud was among the enlightened researchers who theorized that external events might have caused atypical brain function. They looked into their patients' past to find the traumatic event that would explain their current 'madness'.

It follows that through this analytical research into codes of behavior and relationships, general characteristics would emerge within societies that are founded on the basic family unit. This is how researchers were able to create a detailed code of behaviors and emotions that are present in interpersonal relationships.

It is not surprising that these very relationships were recorded 2,500 years ago by ancient Greek tragedians. Indeed their plays provided the nomenclature for the 'complexes' through which psychiatrists of the last century codified human behavior, although everyone now refers to the Oedipus Complex as if it were a discovery that came out of the thorough scientific research of the last century. Yet despite diligent efforts to create a detailed record of the nuances of patients' behavior and expressed and repressed emotions, the etiology of mental illness remains elusive. Even the fictional figure of the schizophrenic mother, who sparked a flurry of excitement among researchers of the 1960s, turned out to be a major fiasco.

Following the accidental discovery of drugs that reduce hallucinations and delusions, as well as other drugs that treat depression, researchers into human behavior were forced to hand the treatment of the mentally ill over to the psychiatrists, who took on the role of the physician, rather than the philosopher and poet. Schizophrenics no longer recline of the psychoanalyst's couch, and patients with depression no longer trawl their past for traumatic incidents, instead they are referred to modern psychiatrists who have been using the appropriate medication to effectively treat psychiatric conditions for decades.

Was all this research on behavior and emotions thrown in the trash along with other great discoveries that were no longer considered useful? Certainly not: this investigation and codification of behaviors, was a response to the impasse in biological brain research in the early twentieth century. It culminated in the resumption of biological psychiatry with state-of-the-art equipment in 1951, having amassed a treasure trove of knowledge, including psychoanalysis, behavioral therapy, cognitive psychotherapy, and all other branches of psychotherapy and theory, which were developed at that time. Initially these theories were limited to mental illness, but eventually they became universal interpretations of human behavior.

All areas of modern life adopted the basic conclusions and the techniques that were developed from these theories. In business they influenced fields as varied as effective leadership strategies, executive recruitment, fostering a team spirit, and product promotion. We now know, for example, that linking the product to sexual desire pays off in increased sales since it has been scientifically established that anything related to the reproduction of the species is strongly attractive.

These theories on mental function can be valuable tools for our daily lives, since each one attempts to explain our behaviors and reactions to the problems that beset us. By better understanding our own processes, we improve our chances of modifying them to our advantage.

This body of knowledge has made a significant contribution to Medicine in general. First of all, Psychiatry has helped consolidate the entire medical community through the role of virtual therapy—the placebo. Drug experimentation has become more credible through the use of double-blind studies, where neither the patient, nor the doctor knows whether they have been given the active ingredient or a placebo. This is necessary to avoid subconscious bias, since research has revealed that it is impossible for this knowledge not to affect expectation and skew the interpretation of the results.

The study of emotions and mental reactions has shown that our mental state is directly related to most of our bodily functions. Anxiety reduces the body's defence mechanisms and can, for example, produce cold sores (Herpes Simplex). It cannot be disputed that depression and stress reduce our immune response, leaving us open to attack by bacteria and viruses. Indeed the effect of our mental state on our overall body function is so vital that it can even extend our lives by a day or two, because of a happy anticipation of a special event.

Our mental state does not only manifest itself through elevated blood pressure when one is stressed, or higher blood sugars when one is sad, but it can also affect the rate of carcinogenesis in our body. It is now believed throughout the medical community that all the body's functions are controlled and coordinated by the brain.

The study and codification of human behavior in the shaping and enriching of clinical practice with more effective models, is another great contribution to Medicine. We now know that for optimum benefits of medical intervention, doctors must allow for the feelings and expectations of their patients. Any treatment is more effective if the patient and their environment are positive. Drugs have fewer side effects, and are far more efficient if the patient is convinced that they are necessary. In contrast, surgery is more likely to present complications if the patient and their environment are negative, and skeptical about the outcome.

This treasure trove of knowledge was developed by Psychiatry during the years when there was no way of carrying our medical biological research of the 'black box'—the human brain. For more than half a century, Psychiatry has been attempting to understand the causes of irrational responses of the brain through the study and analysis of its overall behavior—its responses to stimuli. This was because it had no way of accessing the operation of the circuits inside the 'black box' that resides inside our skulls and dominates us all.

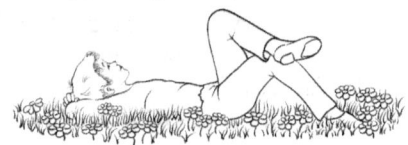

WHAT HAS MEANING IN MY EXISTENCE?

I WAS watching a documentary on TV one day about life in the jungle. At some point the film showed a herd of wild buffalo running to escape a pack of felines, lions or tigers, I do not remember which. It was an impressive scene. There must have been 200 or more buffalo charging in some direction, even they possibly did not know where to, since nowhere did there appear to be any shelter. There were at most ten felines after them, who had already reached the last of the herd, that is, the rear–guard.

The scene was full of suspense and I began to distinguish which one of the last buffalo would first be attacked in one long jump by the wild beasts that by now were dangerously close.

In my ever heretical mind, I thought:

"How dangerous for the poor buffalo, but saving the famished felines. Who knows how long it is since they last fed so richly. They are meat eaters just like us and they need meat. And meat does not grow in the earth nor is cultivated, nor do the delicious hamburgers get to the supermarket shelves from some chemical laboratory."

For carnivores to survive there has always to be some slaughter and violent death. It is a sacrifice of nature for it to reach some species with a better energetic balance such as the flesh–eating animals. Think that the cute little Australian koala as a vegetarian eating only eucalyptus leaves, which have a very small calorific value, has to feed for most hours of its life to survive. So you see that human beings would not be able to create all their civilizations if they were vegetarian and had to be eating all the time just in order to survive.

This is why I considered the sacrifice of the rear–guard buffalo a necessity. Then I had another thought:

"In this hunt the fastest buffalo survive and through that natural selection the buffalo species is improved. The fastest survive and propagate, so they produce little buffalo that can also run faster and have swifter reflexes."

But my doubting mind, that has learned always to question why whatever comes to my notice, saw in the shot of the fleeing herd a lot of buffalo running although they were in the centre. So what? You will ask. Yet, as far as we know, buffalo cannot communicate among themselves. They do not have the capacity of humans to transmit the necessities of nature to all the members of the group. We can therefore say that the last buffalo of the rear–guard are running because they can see the predators approaching. The first ones are running because presumably they saw them first and took flight. But those in the middle, I wondered, why are they running? It must be because all the others are running and they know they have to do whatever the others are doing.

So I think there is some programme in the buffalo's brain that tells them to follow the movements of the group. I also think that this programme is in their brain from birth. It is a protection programme for the animal, to follow the rest of the herd without thinking.

And I wonder also whether perhaps human beings too have such an automatic trigger in their brain. An automatism that makes us run in the direction pointed out to us. All of you will have noticed that we all dash about every day, without really knowing why. So we simply keep running, because the one next to us is running, as well as the one ahead, and the one following and we are afraid that one will take our place if we reduce our pace.

This is why every so often we should stop and reflect, as we humans are more sentient beings than the buffalo of the documentary:

Where are we directing our life to? Whither go we? Is it worth the toil or the effort?

And to take a step further:

As it is a fact that our existence is finite, is our effort perhaps excessive? Do we make plans that correspond to gods and demi–gods and not to ordinary mortals?

What is needed is every so often to do a "zoom–out", as they say in cinema: To put a distance between the focus of our camera and the picture, so as to have a more general overview of the scenery. Not to see only the back of the person in front of us but where the herd is going and reflect whether the direction taken satisfies us. For most of the time we race without knowing what for and to where. Just like the buffalo running in the centre of the herd.

Let us take a personal account of our own life, calmly, let us turn around and take a look back at our history and we will see that most of our decisions were not personally ours. We went to college because we 'had to', for social reasons, to satisfy our parents. Later we were put on a track and chug along like trains, ever faster, competing with those around us and not to satisfy our own necessities. Even what we call our 'necessities' are the result of the influence of others, of fashion, society, our family. Indeed, our personal choices are few. Those are therefore the ones we have to develop.

Let us think of the instant of our final personal judgment, just before we die. That is when they say we balance the accounts of our life. I often pretend I am in a car that leaves the road and plunges at high speed down a cliff. At that instant my whole life unfolds like a film in front of me: The good moments and the bad, the right and the wrong decisions. Were the sacrifices I made worth it? Could I have lived differently? Is it meaningful that I hurt some people and was hurt by some others? Were the efforts I made productive, and my battles? But also, why did I do what I did? Why did I quarrel, why did I leave, why did I go here and there?

I think these two operations, the 'zoom–out' and the 'fast–forward of the film' are the best ways to project a better way of life for us; that is really worth living. Live a life different from that of the herd. Live a life that can on the contrary be an example to others around us who take notice. Not to blindly follow others but guide them on ourselves, in the direction we believe should be taken.

As often as we give ourselves this opportunity to stand back and do a 'zoom–out', so the more consciously do we proceed in our life. We proceed ...we do not follow. This is how we will have the greatest delight at the end of the film of our life. And besides does that not constitute the supreme end (in Greek language the word for the 'end' – 'telos' – has also the sense of purpose).

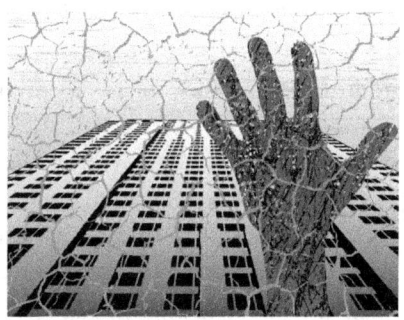

SUICIDE

AS A YOUNG psychiatrist I had undertaken to attend a bipolar (manic-depressive) patient, a Mr P, in the University Psychiatric Clinic. He was a particularly intelligent and cultivated man who had taught at a Boston university for many years. As was also said in the chapter on bipolar disturbance, if patients suffering from this illness, are intelligent and have elements of hysteria in their personality, elements that is that make them strive to be on centre stage and not in the background, have many chances of being successful.

Mr P was hospitalised because he had attempted suicide by overdose. It was his third. He had attempted it twice when he was in the States. All had occurred when he was in periods of depression. In periods of mania contrarily his inhibitions lessened, he spent extravagantly and travelled a lot. He also developed over–sexuality and in some manic phases had extra–marital affairs. In essence he destroyed what he had built during the preceding period. He had already been married twice for this reason, from which he had three children.

In his periods of normalcy, his natural level of functionality was above the norm. He was in what we psychiatrists call hypomania. His brain worked at more 'revs' than the usual. He was very versatile and could reach excesses that led him to have significant discoveries in the field of research to which he was dedicated.

This is the reason for the success of his career despite the false notes he struck, whether in manic phases or in the depressive ones.

So, following the recent attempt, when he had been hospitalised for a few days in the Internal Medicine clinic he was transferred to the University Psychiatric clinic. He was given antidepressant treatment there, at the same time as beginning with lithium as well because of the history of bipolarity, in order to anticipate the phases of the illness.

I was in daily communication with him. It was a contact that from taking his medical history gradually progressed to a psychiatric therapeutic relationship. Mr P had besides, while in America, psychiatric cover of a psychoanalytical type. In the '70s, needless to say, as a distinguished Harvard professor he would have been in psychoanalysis for years. I attempted to bridge this gap in psychotherapeutic communication, under the guidance of course of an experienced psychotherapist.

Besides his exceptional intelligence and brilliance he was a distinguished personage much in the limelight. He had come to Greece two years earlier and had been assigned a post of eminence in applied research. On the other hand, I was but a young psychiatrist. It was therefore easy for me to feel burdened with a heavy responsibility as well as to be delighted to communicate with him. With the guidance of my teacher in psychotherapy I tried to control both sides. Continuing my attendance also after Mr P's relatively brief hospitalisation, I provided psychological support in my private practice too. Exactly because of the complexity of his illness, which from his history showed that it could very easily relapse as well as because of his 'American' habit of regular visits to a psychotherapist, I saw him twice a week.

The history of his illness followed the typical course, one could say, of ever more frequent alternating phases of mania and depression and shorter spaces of normalcy. This will have been and additional and important reason for him to have left the States and returned to Greece. This is where his brothers and sisters and the greater part of his extended family lived, who could if necessary keep an eye on him and give him support.

As Mr P came out of depression my main concern was for him not to relapse into mania but to remain in hypomania, where this particular patient felt well. He was impressively active with his work and professional meetings from the early morning to late at night. It must be said that this enterprise is not at all easy. It is like balancing on a fine thread. At any moment the patient may escape to mania, in a remarkably uncontrolled state. He himself on the other hand, as well his entourage, in no way wished him to be 'regulated' to a lower operational capacity. That is why I found equilibrium, prescribing lithium as a mood stabiliser and a minor dose of an antidepressant.

This entire strategy was, of course, based on our regular contact. In our frequent meetings my patient, habituated to a number of years of psychoanalysis, revealed to me, at the time a young trainee in psychotherapy, that his was an exceptionally interesting person: A man 25 years older than me, with a rich and tumultuous life. It was therefore natural that I should develop sentiments of admiration and see another father figure in him. That is, let us not forget the precepts adopted by Freud, that I transferred to Mr P some of the feeling I had for my father. It was a process I knew and had under control so as not to disturb our basic doctor–patient relationship. On the one hand I ought not to lose respect and have my commands and indications disobeyed. On the other I must not transfer negative elements, which it is natural I would have toward my father, to our relation.

It is another delicate equilibrium, this time on the level of sentiments. Just as in maintaining balance in the illness lithium was of help, in the balancing of our psychotherapeutic relation the supervision of my teacher was of assistance, who helped to keep the balance of the psychotherapeutic dynamics.

If the doctor cannot control the relation with the patient, they should be aware that nearly always the patient will try to 'corrupt' it. It has very often happened to me that patients of mine, mainly of the opposite sex, would try to charm me. If they succeeded, I would no longer be their doctor. I could become just a friend or a lover.

'Corruption' of a relation is frequently attempted by patients, without their being aware of it. It is automatic, because those are the programmes of operation they have in their brain. They try to charm anybody who arouses their interest. They are quite right to do so. But, there are around them some people they should not charm because it will alter some equilibrium of vital significance. The doctor is one of those.

There is not only the sexual side to the chapter on charm, there are many more. Some patients try in an oblique way to display their wealth to me so as to impress me. I remember a woman patient who came to my office with a new expensive handbag every time, which she always placed conspicuously on my desk. Others, in telling their stories will always drop 'important' names, to show they have acquaintances of consequence. There are also others again who try to exert charm with stories of poverty in their childhood or even personal heroic acts.

Therefore the doctor, the psychiatrist in particular, must not in the least be influenced by the charm attacks from their patient. The handling of this attempted charm is decisive in the evolution of the doctor–patient relation. The doctor on the one hand must not be carried away but on the other, they must also not show they reject the patient's offer. The game is played with delicate balancing. That is also why medicine is a particularly charming art to practice!

The patient in question had charmed me, but I think I had managed to stay in control so as to be effective in my role. Two years went by in this way, and from what he said himself as well as from the very few phone calls I exchanged with his companion and his sister, it was something unheard of for Mr P. It was the first time he stayed so well for such a long time: as he was twenty years ago, before his illness; without ups and downs; without enthusiasms and disappointments. Even his character, which had become difficult in the recent past, was somewhat softened.

The second summer came around. We would stop our meetings in August and resume in September. In those days there were no mobile phones for an emergency. My patient would be going to a house in the country with his children, who were grown up by now, who would come from the United States. Afterward, he would then come back to Athens to prepare his work for the new period.

The first week of September passed without his calling me. I must mention here that telephone communication with my patients is never two–way. They know that I shall never ring them to tell them to come to my office. I always consciously leave the initiative to them to contact me, and I make this absolutely clear to them. I do not want them to think I am pressing them so as to have more clients' visits. This is part of my medical code of ethics.

The following week, at about one o'clock the 'phone rang in my office at the hospital. It was the frightened voice of his companion: *"Our friend has killed himself..."* followed by a long silence. I was speechless, frozen. But at the other end there was burning despair: *"I don't know what to do. Doctor, come to the house, please Doctor,"* and she gave me the address.

I was as if under a spell, like a robot automaton. I grabbed my bag and went into the street. I had never before been to his house, which was quite close to the hospital. It was difficult to find a parking space for my car. The narrow street of the block of flats where he lived was blocked by a squad car of the police, who had evidently been called in the meanwhile. I approached and went into the building. My patient's friend who had rung me was at the entrance, in an awful state. His sister stood next to her.

– *Come and see, Doctor... How could such a terrible thing happen?*

We went up to the flat. There was a police officer in civilian clothes at the front door, examining the area. I went into the bedroom. The air was filled with a stench of rotten meat. Involuntarily, I held my nose. Kneeling on the bed, propped on a sporting gun with the barrel in his mouth, was my patient. There were still pieces of his brain sticking to the ceiling and the wall behind him.

I broke out in sweat. I could not stay any longer to behold the sight. I do not remember how I left nor what I said to the friend and the sister. I must probably have identified myself to the security police officer, telling him I was the dead man's doctor and that he had made other attempts in the past.

Never shall I forget the scene nor the abominable smell. The stench of rotten meat pursued me for at least six months. As if a carcass had nested in my skull.

Just as I cannot forget the guilt feelings either that tormented me for a long time. I tried to justify my patient's act... and my failure. My teacher, my guide in the psychotherapeutic relation with my late patient, understood my shattered state and tried to rid me of the guilt.

– *Evidently in August when you went on leave and were not seeing him, the patient had stopped his treatment. His family had also gone away and he will have stayed in town alone. The abrupt interruption of the antidepressants and the lithium brought on depression. Nobody realised it, since he was in Athens alone...*

... Unfortunately you will experience many failures in your medical career. We are not wizards. We are simply counsels of our patients in their illness. Think of surgeons and oncologists. They face defeat every day. That's the way it is. You'll get over it.

I did get over it, only when a month later my patient's friend came to see me at my office. She came unexpectedly. She shook my hand and thanked me for all I had done for that unique person as she put it, and gave me a copy of a small ancient vase that she told me came from an ancient grave found in the Kerameikos. It must be one of those little vials called 'dakryrroi' (tear catcher) in which the Ancient Greeks collected their tears for the dead.

Sadly, in my career I have experienced some other suicides of patients of mine. I have however also had the pleasure of seeing many depressed patients regretting their attempt when after a few days or even weeks of treatment they regained their joy of life. Antidepressant treatment truly makes miracles happen. Sick people who a few days earlier could not only find no meaning to their life but felt so awful that they could not bear it, come back and are grateful to the doctor for having given them life back.

Another thing I often hear from patients suffering from depression, is that not only are they incapable of enjoying anything, but that they also envy those around them who are happy. This is also the reason why one should not press a depressed person to go out and have a good time. Some sufferers after such urging having gone to have fun at some nightclub, wedding, joyful occasion or festivity felt so bad that they thought the only way out for them was suicide. Psychiatrists in the old days noticed that day after a village fête there had been suicides. The villagers would wake up next morning and find somebody had hanged themselves.

There is another truth here: suicides are most frequent in the early morning hours. This is because it is known that in depression, feelings fluctuate over the 24 hours. This means that when the depression is severe, the feeling is worse early in the morning whereas later in the afternoon there might be improvement. There are instances of patients with intense fluctuation of the feeling who say in the morning that they want to kill themselves, while in the evening they go out to a nightclub! This fluctuation is purely biological and is interwoven with the disturbance of biological rhythms observed in depression.

Prevention of suicidal behaviour until the antidepressants take effect is the major problem of the daily practice of psychiatry. The psychiatrist in his office has to evaluate the potential of a patient to commit suicide and give those who accompany them the equivalent instructions.

There are colleagues of mine who do not risk it at all. As soon as they see a manifest possibility of suicide they recommend immediate hospitalization in a psychiatric clinic. There the patient is supposed to be protected from killing themselves. They are supposed to be under constant supervision and, besides, the surroundings of a clinic do not permit acts of desperation. There are bars on the windows, electrical plugs are protected, there are no hooks and pipes from which one could hang oneself and so on, that unfortunately make the clinics like prisons. Many clinics apply extremely strict regulations such as for example not allowing patients to have a razor or even shoe laces.

Despite all these measures, however, the inventiveness of the human brain cannot be foreseen. I shall never forget an incident that occurred in an adjacent clinical unit at some Christmas time, when I was still a resident. A patient managed to choke on a cookie which she crammed down her throat. When the staff realised, it was impossible to remove the cookie crumbs, which had stuck to her larynx. Incidence of suicide may be diminished but never eradicated.

Forcible hospitalisation, but also the voluntary as well, constitute an event of mental trauma both for the patient and for their entourage. This is why I personally follow a more 'heroic' strategy. I try in every way to avoid the sectioning of my patients, which, I assure you, is truly heroic for a responsible doctor.

In fact, so as to substitute to some degree to the security of hospitalisation, I give the patients and their family the security of being in constant communication with the doctor.

First of all I assure the patient, in front of their relatives, that in two weeks at the most they will be feeling much better. I ask for this credit of time to be given me, so as to give the antidepressants the chance to do their work. Of course, initially I base myself on sedative drugs, with use of which I can succeed. Actually, when the anxiety is lessened, depression can better be tolerated by the patient. It seems besides that it is anguish that finally prods the patient to give in to their self–destructive wishes.

I then tell the patient to give me this credit of time although I know depressive patients cannot truly believe they will ever get better.

– I am aware, I tell them, that you think what I am saying is a fairy tale. It is to be expected that depressed people cannot see a ray of light of optimism anywhere. This is besides what depression is. An illness of pessimism. But it is worthwhile to give yourself and me this span of grace, even if only out of curiosity…

The way I say this lets the patient realise that the doctor understands the problem; in general of what it is to be a pessimist. Moreover, they characterise that strange feeling as an illness. In that way the patient sees, perhaps for the first time, that somebody knows about the phenomena that are happening to them. A therapeutic alliance is thus formed, which the doctor can count on to avoid forcible sectioning.

Finally, I involve the patient's relatives and friends in the effort. I tell them that I ought normally to recommend hospitalisation but, that I believe that if they want to help their friend it could be avoided. All I ask them for is to have the patient under constant observation for a few days. In any case, by prescribing an increased dose of sedative medication the patient will stay in bed most of the time. In my experience only very rarely, in cases where the sufferer had a personality problem in parallel with their depression, where those close to them not willing to cooperate.

Naturally, for all the exceptionally 'tied up' and multidimensional approach to suicidal patients, the psychiatrist has a high price to pay of anxiety and responsibility, when they keep a patient out of a clinic. In fact it is often necessary to reassure the relatives themselves and tell them that at any moment they want to, they can take their patient to a clinic. "Clinics are always available". But it is worth the effort to try treatment at home.

Why should I stay alive?

FOR SOME depressed patients, where what they feel can still be changed and has not yet become completely frozen, I try to paint an optimistic scenario for them. Their standard question is: "Why do I have to keep on living? What is the reason to stay alive and go on being tortured?" Quite a lot of patients see no hope anywhere, for any improvement in the objective conditions that led them to depression. A great deal of imagination and inventiveness is needed here. The psychiatrist has to have ready answers and to be practiced in instantly finding untried avenues for the solution of his patients' impasses. True, I acquired this skill in the course of my many years of practicing 'Provocative Psychotherapy', so that I can now easily find a repartee to anything said.

When a lady tells me, crying, that her husband has left her, I answer, joyfully:

– At last! Now you'll be able to find someone who really wants you and will care for you. Because otherwise, you would never dare leave him. That would mean that you would live the remainder of the few, good, years of your only life, in the misery that you and your husband had manufactured for yourselves.

There was also the time when someone in depression told me the bank was going to foreclose on his home and I said to him:

– We see people on TV every day whose houses are destroyed, whether by a fire or a flood or war. A financial crisis is like war. The disasters happen to the undeserving just the same as to the deserving, without being expected and without our having reckoned with them. In wartime, anyone who survived after their home had been bombed were so glad... They may have lost the work of a lifetime, but they think they might perhaps be able to make a life once again. If you had a serious illness, cancer, let's say, everything would be over. But now it's the crisis that has brought about your ruin. As long as you have your health, you will try to build your life up again. And you know what? Your new life may be a better one. After Germany had been razed by the war, nobody expected them to get back on their feet so soon, and especially so much better!

But I cannot forget the occasion when I really could not find words of encouragement to say to a young girl patient. It was the days when the scourge of AIDS was at its peak. No medication against the virus had been found and it meant in practice that anyone suffering from it must not have any more intimate relations with anybody. As a matter of fact, if anyone was known to have it they were completely shunned. There were many instances of employers giving the sack to an employee who was a carrier. Even families adopted the attitude of throwing out one of their members who had it: at that time a father had asked for my help when it was discovered in a blood transfusion test that he was a carrier, with the consequence that his wife had ordered him out of the house so that she and their children would not be infected.

This was then the framework when colleagues at an internal medicine clinic asked me to examine a young woman with AIDS who was contemplating suicide. I did therefore go to see her in her isolating room where she had been hospitalised. I put on a special coat and mask like all the doctors and relatives who visited her, and sat down on a chair next to her bed, I told her what sort of doctor I was, and the young 23–year–old, whose name was Tonia, began telling me her story.

She was a theology student, attending that branch not because it was her choice but because of her school grades. However, theology began to appeal to her in the course of her studies and she planned on graduation to teach religion in high school. While she was a student, Tonia met a young man, a student at the Civil Engineering School. After they had been together for two years and had always made love with a condom, she went on holiday and relaxed, and when she came back to her boyfriend they made love without protection. A few months after she came back, she felt unwell and had tests. She was astounded to be told that not only was she a carrier, she was already ill. It turned out that her boyfriend had had sex with a tourist at the beginning of the summer, by whom he had obviously been infected. He was not ill and had not noticed anything until Tonia's illness was manifested.

What can one say to this poor young woman, when she says she has no reason to live? It is not only feeling betrayed, cheated. It is not only that she will never be close to anybody and will never make love again, not even kiss anyone. Not even her mother, not only a man. It goes without saying that her dream of teaching school disappeared instantly. And, of course, all this for as long as she will manage to survive this life–threatening disease. The sickness had already visibly weakened her and there were clear traces of wounds on her body.

– *What am I to do with this life? Why should I wake up in the morning?*

I admit that I too was overcome. I felt as desperate as she did. I looked around the room and could see no way out. I too wanted to get away from this strangling trap. I happened to look at the window. Mt Hymettos rose in the distance, luminous in the strong Attic sun. I answered her question with something that escaped me, I have to confess, that did sound pompous to my ears and somewhat false, but it was the only thing that came to my mind at that moment:

– *If only to see the sun rise over Hymettos!*

I thought them empty words at first. My voice sounded like a stranger's, but as I thought about it I found they were true. I looked her in the eyes and waited for her reply.

I don't remember what she said but I do remember that we then had a long talk about our existence and our road in this world. I thought I had perhaps given her the reason she wanted to stay alive. When I left the room Tonia's expressive eyes looked at me with gratitude.

That scene was imprinted on my mind as the ultimate limit of despair I could ever confront. Alas, fate did bring me before it again. I faced a similar situation some ten years later.

A young woman, medical student in her last year, had a rare nervous illness that causes progressive paralysis. Within a few months she could no longer get out of bed. Her morale was however brilliant. She did not give up on life. She wanted to have her diploma and asked to be examined in Psychiatry at her home. I have to say I went there with a heavy heart, more out of charity, to do her parents a favour, who had begged me earnestly to go.

I found the young woman in bed, she spoke with difficulty. But I soon saw, to my surprise, that she had really been studying and that she knew more than most of her fellow students. I admired this life's–fighter so much that I wished I could give her something more than the highest marks I gave, because she deserved it. I looked around the room and once more my glance fell on the window, which by coincidence also looked onto Mt Hymettos.

– Please turn her bed around so that every morning she can see the wonderful sunrise.

I said to the parents, wholeheartedly and with the enthusiasm this valiant student inspired me with. This young woman who wanted to hold on to life in every way, reminded me of the desperate theology student.

Suicide is a conscious act of escape, from the unbearable sensation of desperation and of the total incapacity of having any positive emotion. Not having any pleasure in anything must be a particularly disagreeable state. It is tragic not to be able to enjoy anything. I have had patients come to tell me that when now they see their grandchildren, who used to be a delight to them and gave them such joy, because the grandparents are depressed they do not feel anything. They know they should be happy to see them but feel freezing indifference. Wherever they look they see nothing to give them any feeling. They are indifferent to whatever they touch, see, smell – everything. Even their thoughts cannot escape to fly to something joyful. Even their imagination is trapped in indifference.

To go back to my favourite analogy, computers, one could say that depressed patients who manifest a lack of pleasure are like surfing diverse web sites on computer, which however they find empty. Websites the patient expected to find full of enjoyable content are blank. They contain nothing. One can instantly understand the desperation of someone who tries to find a website to interest them and they are all empty or full of indecipherable data. If that happens with our PC it would not be odd if we threw it out. That, precisely, is what the suicidal person does. When they do not find anything in their surroundings that is moving for them, they put an end to their life.

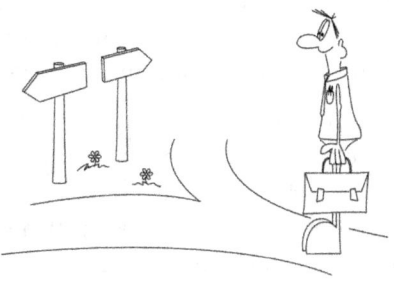

THE PSYCHIATRIST'S MORAL DILEMMA

Antidepressants

NUMEROUS OPPONENTS of antidepressants say that such medicines, especially the latest, which are prescribed with great facility, alter a person's character. This they maintain because they think it something unacceptable and immoral to change a person's character. They are not wrong about the change, but is such a change to be condemned? I often see patients who suffered from depression or anxiety attacks and had taken antidepressants, telling me with joy, years later, that 'they were another person'.

A 28–year–old patient of mine, Eleni, had panic attacks from the time she was a high–school pupil. She had therefore formed a completely superficial sociability. She made friends, boys and girls, but because of her problem could not go with them on all their activities. She could not go out to the cinema or the theatre, nor, later, to bars and nightclubs. She felt uncomfortable in enclosed spaces; she felt a malaise, so she avoided them, giving her friends various excuses.

In this way Eleni acquired an evasive personality, rather phobic. She tried to have friends but she knew that soon, because of her problem, she would have to take her distance, or rather that the others would push her away. As you will expect, her self-esteem was very low, so that she did not go to a tutor's to gain entrance to university level. Her parents were able to have her appointed to a minor administrative position in the civil service. In that office she met a young man who had the same sort of problem and a little later they began a relationship that went on for five years.

The first time Eleni came to my office, she came together with her boyfriend because she could not get around all alone, or rather avoided it because she didn't feel at ease. So her boyfriend had become her permanent escort, just as the girl, because of her friend's similar problem, was in turn his permanent companion.

Anyone seeing them together would however immediately notice how different they were from one another. Eleni was tall and pretty whereas he was a head shorter, his face skin heavily scarred from the acne of his youth. She had a rich vocabulary, he said very little and that was with a strong provincial accent. In a word, they were two people unsuited to each other, obviously linked by the illness.

A few weeks later the medication made its miracle. She felt better and dared to go out alone. She went shopping, went into a cubicle to try clothes on all by herself, without wanting to have somebody she knew waiting outside the curtain. Naturally the next step was to go to a nightclub. But her boyfriend refused to go. Not only would he not talk about such thing, he stubbornly refused treatment. All he would say was typically: "That's how I am. I won't change. Me, I don't like those places — meaning nightclubs, theatres, cinemas and bars, that he disparagingly called 'dives' — to justify his problem, or as is the simple popular saying: 'sour grapes'.

With my encouragement, Eleni went to the cinema, the theatre, even to bars with her girlfriends or her relatives. In the Christmas holidays in fact, the office where she worked organised a dance at a big nightclub and Eleni said she would go.

I leave my mobile phone on, on Saturday evenings, in case my children, who are out, need anything. Only extremely rarely will a patient contravene the rules of polite behaviour and ring me late at night, particularly at weekends. You can therefore imagine my astonishment when I heard Eleni's voice from my mobile at about midnight. There was a lot of background noise and she was shouting:

— *Doctor, I'm in this famous rock star's nightclub, sitting right next to the podium, crushed by hundreds of people. But most of all I feel wonderful. I'm not scared anymore and it's marvellous!*

— *"Good for you!"*

I was shouting too, not only so she could hear me but because I was delighted.

– *And I owe it to you, Doctor.*

– *Have a good time.*

– *Thank you so much…*

The young woman was transformed in a few weeks. From being someone who avoided going out and social contacts she had become a lively and sociable person. Later her relatives were to say that they could not imagine 'their ugly duckling would turn into a swan'. Her boyfriend, who would not take treatment, was the first 'victim' of Eleni's miraculous cure. She left him and from then on enjoyed her independence.

But she did confide in me that she had never felt independent or so self-confident. She had always thought she had a problem. A shy little girl who, when standing up in class to say her lessons, blushed, had sweaty hands and whose throat closed. So she avoided exposing herself to such a state and lived ever more isolated and with ever less self-confidence. She tried to supplement the void in her image by being more diligent in her school work as well as her 'kindness' to others. She never criticised anyone, really because she was afraid of being criticised herself. She became conventionalised with an admirable capacity for tolerating situations.

It may therefore be seen that Eleni's character was formed by her organic problem, which was excessive reaction to stress. Her autonomic nervous system was easily aroused by stress, making her blush and sweat. So she reached the point of being anxious … in case she became anxious. It was to be expected that as a result she avoided potentially stressful situations.

Well, the medication changed that young woman's character, that is to say it gave her the chance to be like 'normal' people. That is how she was rid of her feeling of inferiority that she had had until then. Eleni found her true self. What she could really make of her life and not what her inferiority obliged her to. She broke out at last from the confines imposed by her illness. Yes, this is how Eleni became 'a different person'!

Naturally, as a result of this, her life choices changed, as did the equilibrium she maintained with the persons and the situations around her. Consequently, she was swimming in unknown waters. Of course there is latent danger there. The doctor knows it. As does any parent. But they will trust their child to do well. And the doctor is proud when the patient attains higher levels of functioning.

I too felt pride, trying not to show it, when Eleni, my patient not only made impressive progress at work but also came to my office one day accompanied by an impressive young man. The antidepressants had given Eleni a better chance in life. She was using the gifts God gave her to greater advantage: her good looks and her intelligence. The treatment gave her the strength to get them out of the closet where she had stashed them out shame since she was a little girl.

Therefore, it places the psychiatrist in a moral dilemma when they are enabled by modern medicine to alter a person's behaviour. Should he exercise this capacity? Or is it preferable to let things develop as nature has programmed them? Should we improve people's capacities, since by now technology and human inventiveness give us that possibility?

Many colleagues, mainly psychologists and psychotherapists, maintain that one should not introduce 'chemistry', as they put it, to alter a person's personality. However, 'chemistry', with antibiotics for instance, has saved many lives. Human ingenuity, has helped with spectacles, contact lenses and operation, for us to see better and has improved our natural state. In recent years I have told my patients that were it not for spectacles for presbyopia I would not be able to read, nor of course to write prescriptions. I would have to cease practicing medicine.

This way my patients realise that we utilise 'chemistry' on a daily basis as well as human ingenuity and that we take it for granted. Therefore 'psychoactive–drugs' too are nothing out of the ordinary that we must not use although we have them. It is a human conquest that assists life improvement.

In any case, of course an experienced psychiatrist's judgment and good sense are required,to weigh the conditions existing in the life of every person who asks for their help. They have to calculate the potential of each patient and their surroundings to adjust to new conditions and the 'improvements' they may have to offer. Some become swimmers and swim. For some, alas, it may be too late or, together with their muscular invigoration, swimming lessons be needed.

Improvement with drops

I MAY BE definite about antidepressants and have no moral dilemmas, but I admit to not being quite as categorical about certain other 'psychoactive–drugs'. However, a moral dilemma difficult to solve often arises from the possibility that antipsychotic drugs provide in the containment of a being's behaviour. A minor dose of antipsychotics brings about an alteration of behaviour without other evident side–effects. A short–tempered, assertive or over–active person can become more cooperative and his energies be reduced. A self–centred and autocratic person, with the proper treatment, can feel weakness and as a result become more comprehensive of others.

The alterations of behaviour that antipsychotic drugs are capable of bringing about may be a treatment but also an amputation, depending on the case. This means that if a normal person takes them without psycho–pathology, they will show repression and diminishing of their energy and initiatives. Someone in a manic phase, on the contrary who will of course not accept that their condition is deviatory, with a secret administration of an antipsychotic drug may be brought back to their normal state of mood. It is an intervention that can be the salvation of the patient and of their family too.

I remember the case of a patient, Mr. Nikolas, who was manic. He was about seventy, married, with children and grandchildren. He was a shopkeeper, with a big shop of electrical goods in a quarter of Athens. His relatives told me that he had recently been much more active, slept very little, was on the move all the time, talked more, too much, so that nobody could cut in. He began talking about extending the shop and of opening a chain of stores.

His children, who also worked in the business, had strong reservations. Their father's plans were not based on realistic business plans. They were over ambitious, not to say castles in Spain. But as usually happens, the relatives did not realise this was an illness. It was besides the first time they saw their father in such a state. He had formerly been depressed, but nobody had forewarned them that in the future he could pass to the other extreme of bipolarity.

So his children and his wife were trying to bring Mr. Nikolas 'to his senses'. That is, to dissuade him from his grand schemes by using reasonable arguments. However, of course, all they achieved was to be constantly at odds with the father. Poor Mr. Nicolas on the other hand was on a cloud of bliss and could not understand why his family were preventing him from 'achieving great things'. The state of affairs evolved rapidly. One day, he took the takings of the day and went to the Jaguar representative. He ordered a car that cost way above his means, depositing all the funds he had with him as an advance! Only then did his relatives realise that he was ill.

So they suggested he should see a psychiatrist for an opinion. Mr. Nikolas however would not hear anything about a psychiatrist. He was in seventh heaven, so happy, and saw everything optimistically from there.

– For Heaven's sake, can't I give myself a present? I've been working all these years. It's all my doing. And if I feel like it, in the end, it's my right to destroy it too. It's all mine… But you can see that the time has come to think big. This is my chance in life to take the big step.

He would not listen to reason. He was furious with his wife and children. When they pressed him he said he would go to law to demand his rightful share of the family business and start his own separately. The family came to me in a state of panic.

– The law allows you to resort to the Public Prosecutor to have your man examined

obligatorily by two psychiatrists. If they judge he has to have treatment and he refuses, he will then be taken to a psychiatric clinic by force. There he will be made to take his treatment.

Is what I said to them, and their answer came back from all in unison:

— *And how is he going to go to the psychiatrists for examination? In the state he's in, he won't hear of prosecutors or anything. He's enraged.*

— *The police will come for him, whether he wants it or not.*

— *Policemen and a squad car at our house? Doctor, we have a name in the neighbourhood. Besides, it's our selling point. Imagine him being pulled into the police car and him screaming. It can't be done, Doctor, we will never do that to Dad…*

There was a moment's silence that seemed to us all to last forever. We looked at one another, trying to discern some ray of optimism from somebody's good idea.

When it was all of no avail, I decided to break the silence:

— *In that case, the only solution is for you to try to slip him some medication unbeknownst to him. If that can be done, it might put the brakes on and bring him back to being cooperative.*

They exchanged glances and at once, almost all together, began to ask me what sort of medicine it was, if it would in any way be harmful for him and how it can be administered without his noticing.

A week later of having done this, Mr. Nikolas had calmed down. After a few days he tried to cancel the order of the car, which unfortunately was not possible without the loss of a considerable sum from the amount he had deposited.

His wife, who was responsible for the surreptitious administration of the medication, was in touch with me on an almost daily basis to regulate the dosage. Very soon her husband acknowledged that in the foregoing period he had been in overdrive and had said and done things that were beyond his reasonable self. He had come to what in psychiatry we call normothymia, which means the resumption of the brain's normal rhythm of operation. Neither excessively rapid nor optimistic, as when they are in a manic phase, nor too slow and pessimistic, as when they are depressed. Acknowledging that the state he was in before was morbid, Mr. Nikolas listened to his children when they told him he should consult a psychiatrist. It was thus that he not only understood what had happened to him but to take the treatment that would protect him from a recurrence of the disorder.

It was agreed with the patient's family that he would not be told that the recession of his symptoms had been achieved by a secret medical treatment, and that was for two reasons:

- One, so there would be no possible rift in the trust he had in his wife and sons;

- And second, so as not to eliminate a future possibility of having to repeat the same method of covert treatment. Nobody knows how the situation may evolve in the future. The most cooperative of patients may become fractious and paranoid.

It happens moreover frequently, that patients who have taken their medicine for years without objecting, for some reason, because of what they heard a friend or an 'expert' say, or because they were influenced by somebody, suddenly reduce, or worse, stop their treatment. This is a phenomenon that troubles not only the psychiatrists but the other medical practitioners too. After a heart attack, patients stop smoking for a while and then, when they feel safe, start it again. People tend to forget the difficulties they have been through and to minimise the perils looming in the future. Of course, this is a good defence mechanism to make daily life more bearable and help to dread the future less.

Let us, besides, not forget that the human being must be the only animal that can think and have the mental capacity to be conscious that his life–time is running out. This fact alone could fill them with anguish and be in essence paralyzing him. That is, to lead him to a nihilistic view of everything: since I am going to die, why create anything?

Fortunately, however, for humans, together with the consciousness of their passing lifetime there is also the capacity to shut out that anxiety. So that, in practice, we operate as though we were immortal, what in religion is called 'participation in the divine'. We live our daily life with a prospect of eternity.

But to revert to our story, its moral is that there are times when the doctor must place the good of his patient above the laws and strictures of deontology. They must go back to the old paternalistic practice of medicine, when the doctor had the knowledge and the absolute authority to 'order' a cure. This may, of course, occur only when the doctor has the indisputable outward correct motivation, that he is the true protector of the health of the sick and has no personal gain.

It is unfortunate that in our day the honesty of the practice of medicine has been lost. People are quite right to be suspicious of doctors because doctors too are part of the social system we live in which places personal gain above anything else. When a doctor as well has as his objective the increase of his profits, he loses the prestige of the Priest of Asclepius and he too alas becomes one more craftsman–tradesman. He learned a craft and is trading it.

That is not all. Learning today is not acquired in sanctuaries. It is dispersed all over. Anyone can have access to learning. Anyone can equally claim a false authority and diffuse disinformation all over. This reality obliged us to institute rules of medical deontology and ethics. Rules that oblige us to inform our patients of every medical act we recommend and request his acquiescence before proceeding to anything.

I say the rules are correct for general application but sometimes exceptions may constitute the best solution, as happened in the case of Mr. Nikolas. I think that the good doctor must, in all conscience, be able to overreach the rules and say 'leave it to me', while of course risking the consequences from a society that quite rightly does not encourage heroics and initiatives and the levelling practice making all equal instead.

In the example I have just given, the doctor's moral dilemma may see minor: to follow the rules of deontology imposed on them by the law, or act in the interest of the patient, in essence in contravention of it. There are situations requiring even greater illegality.

A lady called me up one afternoon, who spoke rather hesitatingly and after numerous investigative searching questions asked me if she could come and see me about problems she was having with her husband:

— *It's not our relationship. It's his behaviour in general. Not with me alone.*

— *Come and see me and we'll talk about it together.* And I made an appointment for her at the office.

It was a lady of about forty, quite good looking and well dressed. But in the visit she was just as hesitant as she had been on the telephone. She tried to ask more questions than she gave information. I put her at ease. I did not ask her her name and tried to talk about painless things: how many children she had, if they were boys or girls, if they went to school, if they were good students and other subjects that draw attention away from the problem she really wanted to talk about.

Disorienting questions reduce the anxiety that lies concealed in the focus of interest and facilitate communication. Once more I will say that medicine is a difficult but a fascinating art. It starts out from communication with the patient and, basically, is a question of the doctor's ability to really comprehend the patient.

Very gradually she unravelled her story of pain. Her husband was well off and could provide her with an excellent standard of living. A big house, frequent outings to expensive restaurants, travel abroad for holidays, anything she could wish for. However – and there is always a however, at least for those who come to my office – her husband is very irritable. He quarrels with the domestic staff, he scolds waiters, has misunderstandings with friends and relatives. His behaviour has isolated them socially, although there are always people who keep company with them because of their financial standing and their prominent family name.

She had meanwhile also told me her name.

He was decent with her but was always quick to misconstrue her slightest move. She had realised this and so was careful not to give him occasion to take things amiss. She always told him where she went and let him have complete control of their finances. It was for this besides that on the 'phone she had asked me about my fee. She had been putting aside small amounts in secret, mostly from change, so as to be able to collect the amount of the doctor's fee! For the same reason she had asked if there was waiting time for a visit and how long it would last. She wanted to know how to explain her absence to her husband.

All this I was hearing indeed sounded awful but was absolutely compatible with a diagnosis of a paranoid personality for her husband, something like mild schizophrenia. It appeared from the case history, however, that the man was not so ill as to justify forcible hospitalisation and treatment, that is to say against his will. If therefore the wife applied to the public prosecutor for a forcible examination of her husband it was certain no psychiatrist would sign a forcible hospitalisation order, but that neither could she persuade him to take antipsychotic drugs. He was not doing anything so morbid, nor did he have what in psychiatry we call organised delirium, that for instance for some reason he was being hunted by terrorists or some criminal organisation. He just tended to distort reality very easily and misinterpreted what people around him did and said.

As was detailed in the chapter on schizophrenia, the gentleman evidently had a slight short–circuit in his brain which allows his own reservations toward the environment to enter on the main computer of his brain through the gate whence came the data from external reality. This is why he was convinced that the wariness of his reservations was the absolute reality.

To me it was obvious that for this person to function normally and enjoy his life he ought to be treated with antipsychotic drugs. As obvious was the fact that there was no way the particular patient would accept any treatment whatsoever.

I have to say I felt so sorry for the wife before me, but also for the man himself. Comfortably off as he was, he could have enjoyed a better quality of life. Many people have like him a problem of the brain that makes them live in isolation and grumbling. They are people we call 'friendless', they are anti–social, quarrelling and finding fault with everybody; people who are easily annoyed and pick a fight. Mostly, of course, with those close to them, because they are an easy target it will not have serious consequences, but also with those they work with, or even third persons.

I therefore risked proceeding with what is according to the rules of deontology, to an 'immoral' or, more, 'illegal' act: I told her that the only way I could see for her possibly to find a way out from the situation was, undetected, to slip him some antipsychotic drug. I explained the problem her husband must have, according to what she had told me, as well as the manner in which I had hopes the medicine would improve it.

The lady did not hesitate. She agreed immediately, to the point that I thought she had maybe come to see me with the plan already in mind. I began to have second thoughts, more cunning. Did she perhaps have an idea of repressing him to such an extent through the treatment as to make her husband more easily manageable? Did she want to make him her puppet? My mind started concocting scary scenarios. The medicine I had in my hand could become poison. Because of course the doctor has to take action always in the interest of the patient. Not to harm him.

I went on to make a scrupulous estimate of the motives of the lady I had before me. I tried to see if there would be any manifest benefit for her beyond the improvement in his conduct. Finally, I trusted my instinct. I judged her to be innocent. She seemed to have had a bad time but also to be decided to stay with her husband, from whom she knew she had been given a fine lifestyle, financially and socially.

So I proceeded to write out the prescription for the antipsychotic drugs that I had suggested she administer secretly to her husband without, obviously, his knowledge. I did feel a schemer and conspiratorial, but as usual I looked on the bright side. I asked her to be in touch with me again soon so as to tell me of developments. I realised, of course, it would not be easy since her husband kept such a tight check on what she spent, on her time, and, possibly, on her phone calls.

Notwithstanding, the lady managed to make contact with me a month later. I had been consumed with anxiety all that time. Was I the good wizard or the crafty accomplice in a crime? Once again she made a lunchtime appointment and came in to tell me the news.

It was good news. The husband was becoming more compliant and less irritable. She looked perfectly happy, she was glowing. She was not a bad person, and that reassured me. She wanted to talk about her new way of life.

— *Two days ago a waiter accidentally stained his clothes. I expected a big scene and that as usual we would become a spectacle. I was astonished, because my husband reacted very mildly. In fact a friend of mine who was with us that evening and who knows us very well, said the next day she had been impressed by my husband's sangfroid… Doctor, we are getting on very well. Thank you very, very much. I should have come to see you earlier.*

— *Don't get carried away. The results may show that your husband needed pharmaceutical treatment, but you can't slip it to him behind his back for ever. We shall have at some point to persuade him to take it himself. In a gentle way said, when he is more cooperative, you have to convince your husband to come and talk to me. I don't know what excuse you'll find, perhaps not his bad temper, maybe headaches, stress, depression, sleeplessness. Only when I can finally persuade him to take some medicine on his own, will we be able to say: mission accomplished.*

She kept coming back every month, to tell me of her continuing successes. The husband was now completely cooperative. He was however beginning to be a 'heavyweight'. He slept a lot and did not much want to go out or go on trips. It looked as though the dose was excessive. The clever wife, always bearing in mind what I had said, persuaded him to visit me so as to give him something to shake him up a bit, what we call 'boost' him.

Our secret scheme worked perfectly. The husband came, supposedly recommended to do so by a friend of his wife's who had spoken of me. It was true, with the treatment his wife was giving him on the side, as he told me he was feeling flaccid, sluggish. I took the opportunity this gave me to propose a pill that contains a little antidepressant as well as a small quantity of antipsychotic medicine, that I calculated would keep him away free of the irritability and paranoid inclination of the past.

I must have gained his trust. For some months, at least for a few months when I was in touch with his wife, he was taking his medication by himself and all was well. If that had been the end of the story, I would have been pleased with myself. The moral lesson would have been once again that the transgression of deontological rules, well–meaning, in the best interests of the patient, by a doctor who had good intentions had been absolutely justified. However, there is more to the story…

When the summer was over, about a year after the lady's first visit to my office, she came to see me again. She now felt very familiar with me and she opened her heart to me. She confessed to having had an extra–marital affair for a number of years. The man was of their circle, married, with a family and two children, older than hers. She did not reveal his name, but did tell me he was even better off financially than her husband.

I listened, as indifferently as I could, trying not so much as to blink. I was thinking that there was in front of me what is called a femme fatale. A woman who not only married a very rich man and lived a life of luxury, but who was able to manipulate him, tricking a psychiatrist, and here she was now telling me she has caught an even wealthier man in her nets! As she talked, I was thinking this was not a female to be toyed with.

But a psychiatrist's job is never boring. While I was becoming certain that I had a monster to deal with, the lady was gradually transformed into a harmless being who needed protection and care. She confided to me that eight years after her marriage, when she was aware of her husband's problem and the Calvary she had ahead of her, she had met his gentleman. They had stayed with him, her and her husband and her children, who were then little, at his chalet in Switzerland for New Year's Eve celebrations. He must have been enchanted as soon as he met her and tried to get close to her every way he could.

— *I was flattered, but there was no way I could ever dream of giving in to his constant and pressing attentions. Maybe I felt I was condemned to spending the rest of my life with a particularly difficult man, but I had two small children and I could not imagine anything else... But he was very insistent, and my husband on the other hand... it was as if he did everything to push me into the other's arms. He was becoming ever more abrupt, showing me and the children more hardness all the time. He yelled, was annoyed, quarrelsome, every day more domineering. While the other one rang me up every evening to say goodnight... his voice sounded so calm and sweet to me that it was as if he was a soporific, which I was certainly beginning to need after a day spent under the pressure of my husband all day.*

She took a deep breath. She seemed to be suffering and tears came to her eyes. Having done this work for so many years, I know now when the tear ducts get the message from the brain. The eyelids flutter more rapidly and stay closed a little longer. Breathing gets slightly deeper and slower. The throat closes and gulps, trying in vain to swallow.

Before the storm breaks, the brain coordinates certain functions. It isolates itself from exterior circumstances and focuses its thoughts on here it is in pain. It digs at a certain point until the tears drop. Depending on the intensity of the feelings, sometimes a timid drop flows and sometimes, as if the digging struck an artesian vein, tears flow abundantly, with sobs.

— *I resisted as long as I could, but my struggle was hopeless. We were invited to spend a week skiing at his chalet. I tried to get my husband to refuse to go, but, as always, he wanted the opposite of what I did... Anyway, that gentleman and I had an affair that has lasted the past three years. He gave me what I lacked, tenderness and affection. He stood by me and endured all my husband's eccentricities. It was very difficult for us to meet. My husband's jealousy made us find the most incredible subterfuge. That was yet another nightmare for me. I say for me, because I didn't want my husband to have the slightest suspicion. There was no way I was going to divorce. On the other side, the other man was relaxed. He would say: "Don't be scared. If he finds out about us, you'll leave him and I will definitely marry you. I'll divorce my wife and we'll get married."*

Yeah, I thought. That's what they always say; big words and promises. And when the time comes: "We'll see... it isn't easy, my wife won't give me a divorce", and other excuses. I have come across plenty of such instances in my career.

— *... However, after you came onto the scene and my husband was treated, he began to be once again the lovable person he was when I first met him, and I felt the other guy was completely redundant. I do love my husband and even what little he gives me now is quite enough for me. He isn't sharp with me, he listens to my opinion. He's companionable and he's nice to the children...*

The other man on the other has become dangerous. The more I try to keep a distance from him the more he tries to make my position difficult. He suddenly appears in front of me unexpectedly. The other day, my husband and I were having dinner in a fashionable restaurant with friends and he suddenly came in with his wife. As he said, someone he knew, who was with us, told him where we were and he turned up. I have asked him to break it off but, he won't hear of it. If I insist he threatens to tell my husband about our affair...

Again she breathed deeply. She looked at me keenly and went on with the flood of her confession.

– *He's mad. Doctor, you have to save me. You gave me and my family happiness, you have to do something to get me out of this nightmare.*

But the relief was that I was coming out of my nightmare at that moment! Fortunately for me, that lady was not sly and evil as I had feared for a moment. She had not used me for her underhand plans. It appeared she had genuinely wanted her husband cured and not to exploit him. She did not want to neutralise him, she wanted him to improve.

This however taught me a lesson. Psychopharmacology gives me enormous power, but exceptional prudence is needed in its utilisation. It is only too easy to employ such power with the wrong objective.

In this particular case, the only advice I could give her was to cease every contact with the other man. Not to answer any of his messages and, of course, never accept to meet him again. All of it of course when she will have very calmly explained the state of affairs to him, and that there was no possible way she would see him again. As for his threat of telling the husband all, I told her to stress that if he did such a thing it would only make him hateful to her and even more frivolous than she thought him now. Not more loving. His mania to bring her back to him was just like the fury of a child when a toy is taken away from it.

This was also to be our last meeting. I do not know what happened next. All I know is that she did not divorce, because if she had I would have heard of it from society circles, because as I have said, her family was very well known. I hope that she will not use the know–how I gave her in the use of antipsychotics for any bad purpose.

Advice on eugenics

A FATHER brought me his son, Theodore, 32 years old, a school–teacher at a school near Athens. In the past month Theodore had been uneasy and was having intense delusions. He thought his pupils were the same he had been teaching years earlier when he was a teacher in his native village in a northern province. He thought they had changed their names and were wearing different clothes so as to confuse him. A few days before he had made a scene in class, demanding that his pupils tell him the reason for this 'game', and the headmaster, who must have realised Theodore's mental problem, had given him a month's leave.

After trying for a long time, I managed to persuade Theodore to take antipsychotic treatment. Sure enough, a few weeks later he had calmed down and was facing the prospect of returning to his school, albeit with some reservations, generally with optimism however. Back at the school, the headmaster did not of course entrust a grade to him but kept him busy with clerking work. Theodore was suspicious of the students but no longer thought they were playing a trick on him.

– *They are the same, Doctor... but now they're not being provocative, as they were a month ago.*

– *You see that being calmed by the medication now you see things with greater composure?*

– *No, I don't think the medicine has anything to do with it. I think the pupils and their parents got the message that I'm on to them, so they stopped playing games with me.*

The school term came to an end. Then, however, Theodore decided to cease taking his medicine, with the result that the next term he had the same symptom as before. This time he did not declare his delusions openly. Urged by his parents, he came to see me again and from then on he accepted to take his treatment all the time.

So, not only could he do his job, that year and the next, but two years later he announced that he had got married! And oh my goodness, what's more! It seems the spouse too had some mental health problem because she too was not sociable and they had met through their parents' match-making.

It has been seen that what parents of schizophrenics desire above all is to marry them off. They think in that way they will be relieved of the great burden of dealing with the illness. They hope the burden will be shifted onto the shoulders of the spouse. In fact I have often heard those poor parents say: "*What is going to become of our child, when we are gone?*" "*For our child, marriage would be security.*"

In this anguished effort to 'see their child settled' parents generally try to conceal the existence of a mental problem. Even if it comes out, they try to hide the person's need for constant and conscientious pharmaceutical treatment. Trying to gloss over their child's defect presenting it as minor as possible, they usually say he or she once had a 'slight' nervous breakdown or a 'nerve storm'. But now they are just fine! And of course it goes without saying, absolutely no need for medication.

There is however nothing more deceptive than having 'provided for' the sick child under such conditions. It is if they were leading them to certain relapse. It is not only the stress of the wedding and the changed circumstances of the patient's habits. Even before their wedding, on outings and excursions, patients will neglect taking their medicine scrupulously. They either have them with them and take them secretly when they can or, worse, they do not take them along at all so as not to be discovered.

It is however after marriage also that parents, who supposedly fulfilled their duty and breathe a sigh of relief, encourage the patient to stop the treatment, "… since you're fine now and you don't need the medicine any more". It is an almost mathematical certainty that even the wedding preparations will lead all schizophrenic patients to relapse.

For this reason, and overcoming any moral qualms or dilemma, I am by now directly opposed to marriage of schizophrenics. I have seen very few exceptions when a schizophrenic has been able to maintain a satisfactory marital relationship. In these rare cases, too, the marriage was based on absolute sincerity.

To revert to Theodore's case, not only did he get married, and in fact to all appearances to another schizophrenic, they also proceeded to have a family. Five years later he came to tell me that he already had two children. Unfortunately, both of them had problems. The elder could not yet speak, although he was four, and the baby, according to specialists who were seeing it, was autistic.

Theodore was treating this frightful drama not only absolutely calmly, it may be said, even superficially. He divorced his wife and left her to deal with the enormous problem alone, fortunately with the help of her parents. He himself retired, and was now free to look for another wife!

Theodore's case is typical and contains two great moral dilemmas. The first concerns whether a schizophrenic is in a condition permitting him to get married. And the second concerns his having children.

On both these points, Psychiatry has not taken a clear stance. Most psychiatrists, including myself in the early years of my career, are in favour of encouraging patients to complete their socialisation through marriage. For it is true that a marital relationship, a close relation of companionship as it develops in a marriage may be considered as the fulfilment of a person's sociability. Consequently, in the effort to increase the functionalism of a schizophrenic, most psychiatrists encourage them to marry, or at least in numerous instances, will not dissuade them from marriage.

But after marriage, of course, the question of bearing children or not arises. There again, many psychiatrists simply compare figures. The chances of a schizophrenic having a schizophrenic child are about 14%. If, however, both parents are schizophrenic the possibilities rise to 40%. It is a percentage frequent in such marriages, since, let us not forget, both sides usually conceal their illness. Our patient thus speaks for and calculates for himself but is often unaware that on the other side there are also a number of pathological genes.

However, having said this, what meaning does a dry percentage–figure have? What, in the end, interests whoever asks for genetic advice is to ensure they will not have a child with a problem, that they will not bring themselves a 'cross' to be borne for a lifetime.

Well, then, 14% is a huge percentage. It is ten times greater than the average for the general population, that is, all of us. That is why it is totally irresponsible for a psychiatrist to encourage a schizophrenic, already 'disabled' to embark on such an adventure. I believe they should do everything to dissuade them, both the patient as well as their parents.

There arises here an even more fundamental quandary. Until about 60 years ago when antipsychotic drugs were discovered, all patients suffering from schizophrenia were obliged to spend their life either in asylums or lived marginal lives in the little communities of their native place. They were what everyone called 'the village idiot'. In some cases it could even happen that they lived imprisoned in some basement so that nobody would find out, which would stigmatise the entire family. There were, moreover, and sadly there still are, a number of cases of schizophrenics who are jailed because of a crime committed, most probably in a delirious state, but for whom nobody has bothered to have a diagnosis and the specialised treatment. They are left to spend their years in prison like common criminals, without the specific care the law provides for such cases.

Nowadays, exactly because of and thanks alone to pharmaceutical treatment, these sufferers circulate amongst us, and what's more without our noticing them. As long as they take their medication they function in an almost normal way. There are also cases, in fact, where the brain damage is minor and also the treatment was initiated in time, where functionality remains exceptional. The result is that these patients reach the point of claiming the right to have children.

This is why the psychiatrist, who has the knowledge, but particularly because they have the medicine in their quiver that bring the increased functionality, is also the one who has to draw the patient's attention to the consequences of child–bearing. It is modern Psychiatry which has brought the patients into the dance of proliferation of our species, whilst the illness had taken them out of it. This means that the frequency of the illness will increase in the generations to come. It is something that, if seen for the angle of eugenics, is extremely unfavourable for our evolution.

The counter–argument is obviously that Medicine in general, thanks to the leaps of advance it had made in the past decades, has reversed the role of natural selection. It keeps within the dance of multiplication many persons with a diseased constitution who would not normally reach the age of fertility or, if they did, would not be targets for selection by the opposite sex.

It is my hope that these dilemmas will be solved by Medicine when, in the near future, it will make progress in genetic engineering, when, that is, it will enable us to have descendants according to our wishes, custom–made, on order. Then too, of course, it will be the end of Evolution as we know it to this day. We will then take the driving seat of pre–planned evolution, where Man will take the place of God at the wheel of Evolution. I hope that until that moment mankind's inner cultivation will have given them so much wisdom that they will not singe their fingers with matches like the boy playing with fire.

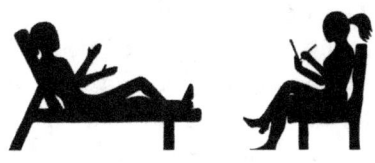

PSYCHOANALYSIS: AN ATTEMPT TO CHANGE A BASIC PROGRAMME

THE TRAGIC state of the ineluctability of human behaviour when the earliest models have been imprinted makes one think of Fate. It means that one's choices are not made freely but obey to the models 'built–in' to each person's mind.

Everything seems to have been pre–ordained and fated. From the simplistic: I choose my wife because she resembles my mother (in appearance, colour of her eyes, or her character or the over–protectiveness she shows me), to my choice of profession, as well as my behaviour toward my children. A human being is a blind Oedipus who leads a life determined by his fate, by the character he formed in the first years of his existence.

Psychoanalysis has come to liberate mankind from such a fate. Classic psychoanalysis is a therapeutic technique, in which the person treated – whom here we shall call 'the patient'– lies on a sofa for about 45–50 minutes at a time, 4–5 times a week, and talks. They talk freely about whatever they want, whatever comes to their mind. The therapist – that is the analyst – is behind them or next to them but where he or she cannot be seen. The analyst remains mute. They do not give answers. Their only concern is to promote the monologue, which is to say the spoken discharging of 'the patient'.

Initially the monologue seems to be addressed to the analyst. However, in due course, when 'the patient' realises they will not have a reply, they will begin speaking as if it were to their self. This is also reinforced by what is known as 'free associations'. From the start the analyst encourages 'the patient' to say anything that comes to mind, as far as possible avoiding any critical thought and the censorship of logic, like surfing the Web of their brain– with no objective.

For this to be attained, it goes without saying that first of all complete confidentiality on the part of the analyst has been ensured. Furthermore, it is necessary for the analyst not to exercise any critique on what 'the patient' says. And believe me, this is hard, because 'the patient' will try in every way they can to have a reply to that they are saying. They seek the confirmation or rejection from the analyst, whom they see as a parental figure. Despite the provocation, the analyst must not only avoid saying: 'you said some good things today', 'you're right', they must also not allow any sign of external communication to show: a sympathetic look or a nod of acquiescence, a reassuring pat on the back or as much as a warmer handshake on saying goodbye. The analyst has to be emotionally frozen and distant, while at the same time in some way showing their interest in the monologue of 'the patient'. The 'patient' must have the impression all the time that behind them there is somebody eager to follow them as they surf their mind, and that through this surfing they will be led, under their own power, to their Ithaca. That is to say in a state wherein they will think, and especially, act differently, released from the fate that repeatedly led them to make the same mistakes.

During this entire Odyssey, the analyst is following and encouraging. The only instrument they are permitted to utilise is interpretation and to remind of similar situations in the past. To intervene, that is, in some account of 'the patient' 'Ulysses', interpreting his positive feelings for 'Circe' as being due to her resemblance to the mother. Or to remind the traveller, if he has found another enchantress like the sorceress Circe, what happened last time with a witch like her.

Using these reminders as a tool, the analyst influences 'the patient' not to repeat the same errors, interpreting their behaviour as deriving from their basic programming, which to say their fate, from which they seek to escape. They will point out the tendency 'the patient' has of repeatedly following the route they know, since this route too, if taken again, will lead them to the familiar outcome which, as they declared at the outset, they wish to avoid.

In this way, what the person being analysed does is to try to manufacture fresh avenues of behaviour in his mind. As a matter of fact, in order for these new routes to be preferable to the old ones trodden before, they have to be trodden many times. That is to say they must be employed repeatedly, so as in time to become their preferential routes. It is of course to be expected that initially the selection of the new path does not happen automatically. It is the result of conscious planning, so as to avoid the erroneous automatically triggered patterns of behaviour.

It is the person analysed who has to have the choice of planning the new course, which is why the analyst's role has to be a passive one. They must not be the one to indicate the direction, all they have to do is point out the mistakes in the planning of the route: *"This way, as you know from experience, leads you to the conduct which, as you yourself have said, you want to avoid."*

The analyst's passivity plays yet another significant role: 'the patient' does something, or refers to something from their past, or speak of their intention for the future, awaiting a reaction, such as they received from their father or mother.

As an example, when I was growing up I was thin and was pressed to eat more. My mother was always running after me with a forkful, trying to stuff me. I therefore tell my analyst that I have recently lost my appetite, in fact, have lost some weight, and that this scares me that I am heading for anorexia nervosa. I think my analyst will react to what I say or do in the same way as my mother did in a similar situation and will urge me to eat. In this way in the place of my analyst I shall see my mother. This is what is called 'transference'.

If, however the analyst, as they should, restrain themselves and do not react, I shall then say to myself: What's going on here? Here I am losing weight, and s/he doesn't care? It isn't at all like my mother, with whom, every time I wanted her attention, I just had to refuse my food. This is how I was forgiven other misdemeanours, or I did get her attention, away from my sister or my father. It meant of course that I was a skinny little boy and felt rather inferior to the other boys in my grade at school.

Now, when I cannot touch my analyst with my 'anorexia', I come to realise that the behaviour is useless. And I also realise what the problems in the image I presented to others were, and, consciously, I begin to eat.

The analyst's passivity – the reaction from them I do not expect – makes me seek other ways to push his buttons than those I knew, which were, that is, fresh in my repertoire. And so I fabricate fresh prototypes to arouse the interest of the important people I have around me.

What matters is that these fresh repertoires should be more easily accessible, or shall we say, more ready, to hand, for me to resort to them at the first opportunity, instead of to the old ones, that may be familiar but are now condemned. The answer to this requirement is given, in classic psychoanalysis, by the frequency of repetition of the new repertoires.

The new short-cuts and the new programmes that the analysed persons themselves have made in their brain's computer are repeated and, eventually, take the place of the 'favourite' programmes and consequently the old 'favourite' programmes decline in popularity, falling to the worst places on the scale.

Psychoanalysis is a difficult and slow process, the efficacy of which depends on many factors. Most important is the motivation of 'the patient' but equally so is the ability of the analyst. Above all, however, what must be understood is that never, ever does it treat the illnesses that psychiatry is called upon to deal with. Psychoanalysis attempts to smooth dysfunctional behaviour patterns and moreover, to substitute them with other, more adaptable and successful behaviours. In that way it succeeds sometimes to make a life more bearable, less mentally wearying, easier and more agreeable. It assists in avoiding pitfalls and deleterious ventures that had brought mental distress. It tries to alter the keyboard of our brain's computer, to make it more ergonomic, to accord with fresh needs and aspiration. It is in other words a method that may sometimes alter the course of a life and extract us from the one-way street where all seems to be predestined and fated.

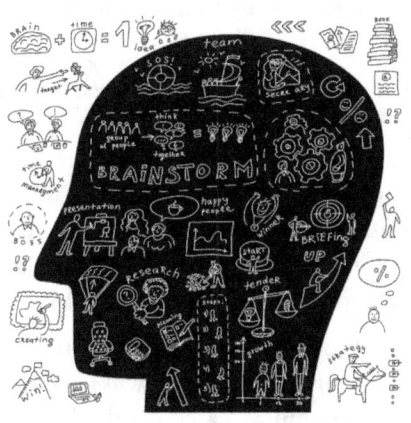

IN LIEU OF AN AFTERWORD: PSYCHIATRY AND RATIONALISM

DOCTORS are nowadays very often carried away by the dizzy technological evolution to be seen all around and indeed inundating their work, to the extent they think they are exercising a technological profession. What our surgeon colleagues want, for example, is a better topographic imagery of the damage and a more exact method of approaching and cross–sectioning. They are therefore very well–satisfied with the modern methods of detailed imagery of the various body parts offered by MRI and its daily improvements. On the other hand, the machinery of robotic surgery gives them the opportunity to see their operational field ten times enlarged, so as to effect incisions with absolute precision, thus neutralising the slightest tremor of their hand.

However, even surgeons need to persuade their patients to trust them. Furthermore, surgeons also need to provide psychological support to their patients subsequently too in the hard task of the healing process. It is a process, as we psychiatrists know only too well, that also depends on the patient's psychological state as well as on their attitude to their illness, their doctor and the entourage, both of the family as well as the social milieu.

Even those technocrats of health have to know the optimum manner in which to announce unpleasant diagnoses to their patient, as well as to deal with the anguish of the relatives. Every time, they too have to calculate the cost and the benefit that will arise from their every intervention on the patient. Even they have to be able to enter psychologically in the place of the patient, that which we psychiatrists call 'empathy'.

And if this is valid for a 'technical' specialisation such as surgery, how much more does it go for psychiatry! It may be becoming daily more 'biological', that is that progressively the biological base upon which our behaviour is 'imprinted' is revealed, however we also perceive the influences this base and its functions receive from the surroundings. We recognise the imprints that are there from birth, that were imprinted when that base was still soft and malleable, as well as those imprinted at a later stage and which are the 'habits' of adult life.

Therefore, just as for other medical specialisations, psychiatry, nevertheless, thanks to its tremendous biological evolution, will never become dry technology. Nonetheless, the progress made in research on the brain obliges us to abandon the philosophical notions about the formation of human behaviour. To the layman, terms may sound highly interesting such as 'introjection of aggression as pathogenesis of depression', but even the last medical student knows today about certain serotonin brain circuits that are malfunctioning.

The time has come for psychiatry to cast off the cloak of metaphysics that brought it closer to Philosophy and Theology, and for it to concentrate on prosaic and measurable biological research. As it matures, Psychiatry abandons unbridled imagination and restricts itself to rationalism.

I am aware that as a process, for some 'colleagues' this is particularly painful. They cannot however continue to obstruct progress and, especially, sell those dreams of their fantasy about a Science, for quite simply, it is not a science. They are illusion of the past that have by now become part and parcel of the History of Medicine. I believe that if this book is of any assistance it is in precisely this direction. To bring release from the myths that accompany Psychiatry and, unfortunately, continue to plague people. With the aid of modern biological research on the brain, Psychiatry has decoded many of the 'mysteries' that gave rise to thousands of prejudices and made mental illnesses 'divine', 'magical' and 'accursed'.

www.ingramcontent.com/pod-product-compliance
Lightning Source LLC
Chambersburg PA
CBHW070121110526
44587CB00017BA/2877